New Frontiers
in the Study of
Gene Functions

NEW HORIZONS IN THERAPEUTICS
Smith Kline & French Laboratories Research Symposia Series

Series Editors: George Poste and Stanley T. Crooke
Smith Kline & French Laboratories, Philadelphia, Pennsylvania

DOPAMINE RECEPTOR AGONISTS
Edited by George Poste and Stanley T. Crooke

MECHANISMS OF RECEPTOR REGULATION
Edited by George Poste and Stanley T. Crooke

NEW FRONTIERS IN THE STUDY OF GENE FUNCTIONS
Edited by George Poste and Stanley T. Crooke

NEW INSIGHTS INTO CELL AND MEMBRANE TRANSPORT
    PROCESSES
Edited by George Poste and Stanley T. Crooke

New Frontiers in the Study of Gene Functions

Edited by

GEORGE POSTE *and*
STANLEY T. CROOKE

Smith Kline & French Laboratories
Philadelphia, Pennsylvania

PLENUM PRESS • NEW YORK AND LONDON

Library of Congress Cataloging in Publication Data

New frontiers in the study of gene functions.

(New horizons in therapeutics)
Includes bibliographies and index.
1. Gene expression. 2. Genetic regulation. 3. Microbial genetics. 4. Genetic
engineering. I. Poste, George. II. Crooke, Stanley T. III. Series. [DNLM: 1. Genetic
Intervention. II. Genetics, Biochemical. QH 450 N532]
QH450.N5   1987   575.1   86-30313
ISBN 0-306-42502-5

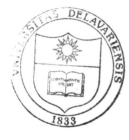

© 1987 Plenum Press, New York
A Division of Plenum Publishing Corporation
233 Spring Street, New York, N.Y. 10013

Printed in the United States of America

Contributors

Richard Axel, Howard Hughes Medical Institute, College of Physicians and Surgeons, Columbia University, New York, New York 10032

John Brady, Laboratory of Molecular Virology, National Cancer Institute, National Institutes of Health, Bethesda, Maryland 20892

Michael R. Briggs, Department of Biochemistry, University of California, Berkeley, California 94720

Ana B. Chepelinsky, Laboratory of Molecular and Developmental Biology, National Eye Institute, National Institutes of Health, Bethesda, Maryland 20892

Leonard Chess, Department of Medicine, College of Physicians and Surgeons, Columbia University, New York, New York 10032

Paul R. Clapham, Institute of Cancer Research, Chester Beatty Laboratories, London SW3 6JB, England

Deborah Cowing, Department of Bacteriology, University of Wisconsin, Madison, Wisconsin 53706

Angus G. Dalgleish, Institute of Cancer Research, Chester Beatty Laboratories, London SW3 6JB, England

Benoit de Crombrugghe, Laboratory of Molecular Biology, Division of Cancer Biology and Diagnosis, National Cancer Institute, National Institutes of Health, Bethesda, Maryland 20892

Janet Duvall, Laboratory of Molecular Virology, National Cancer Institute, National Institutes of Health, Bethesda, Maryland 20892

Beverly M. Emerson, Laboratory of Molecular Biology, National Institute of Diabetes, and Digestive and Kidney Diseases, National Institutes of Health, Bethesda, Maryland 20892

James Erickson, Department of Bacteriology, University of Wisconsin, Madison, Wisconsin 53706

Gary Felsenfeld, Laboratory of Molecular Biology, National Institute of Diabetes, and Digestive and Kidney Diseases, National Institutes of Health, Bethesda, Maryland 20892

Anne Ferguson-Smith, Department of Biology, Yale University, New Haven, Connecticut 06511

Gerald R. Fink, Whitehead Institute for Biomedical Research, Massachusetts Institute of Technology, Cambridge, Massachusetts 02142

Martin Gellert, Laboratory of Molecular Biology, National Institute of Diabetes, and Digestive and Kidney Diseases, National Institutes of Health, Bethesda, Maryland 20892

Maurice Godfrey, Department of Medicine, College of Physicians and Surgeons, Columbia University, New York, New York 10032

Carol Gross, Department of Bacteriology, University of Wisconsin, Madison, Wisconsin 53706

Alan Grossman, Department of Bacteriology, University of Wisconsin, Madison, Wisconsin 53706

Charles P. Hart, Department of Biology, Yale University, New Haven, Connecticut 06511

Michael H. Hecht, Department of Biology, Massachusetts Institute of Technology, Cambridge, Massachusetts 02139

Joanne E. Hesse, Laboratory of Molecular Biology, National Institute of Diabetes, and Digestive and Kidney Diseases, National Institutes of Health, Bethesda, Maryland 20892

P. David Jackson, Laboratory of Molecular Biology, National Institute of Diabetes, and Digestive and Kidney Diseases, National Institutes of Health, Bethesda, Maryland 20892

Rudolf Jaenisch, Whitehead Institute for Biomedical Research, Massachusetts Institute of Technology, Cambridge, Massachusetts 02142

James T. Kadonaga, Department of Biochemistry, University of California, Berkeley, California 94720

Kamel Khalili, Laboratory of Molecular Virology, National Cancer Institute, National Institutes of Health, Bethesda, Maryland 20892

Jaspal S. Khillan, Laboratory of Molecular Genetics, National Institute of Child Health and Human Development, National Institutes of Health, Bethesda, Maryland 20892

George Khoury, Laboratory of Molecular Virology, National Cancer Institute, National Institutes of Health, Bethesda, Maryland 20892

Frank A. Laski, Department of Biochemistry, University of California, Berkeley, California 94720

Catherine D. Lewis, Laboratory of Molecular Biology, National Institute of Diabetes, and Digestive and Kidney Diseases, National Institutes of Health, Bethesda, Maryland 20892

Michael R. Lieber, Laboratory of Molecular Biology, National Institute of Diabetes, and Digestive and Kidney Diseases, National Institutes of Health, Bethesda, Maryland 20892

Dan R. Littman, Howard Hughes Medical Institute, College of Physicians and Surgeons, Columbia University, New York, New York 10032

Paul J. Maddon, Department of Biochemistry and Molecular Biophysics, College of Physicians and Surgeons, Columbia University, New York, New York 10032

Kathleen A. Mahon, Laboratory of Molecular Genetics, National Institute of Child Health and Human Development, National Institutes of Health, Bethesda, Maryland 20892

J. Steven McDougal, Immunology Branch, Centers for Disease Control, Atlanta, Georgia 30333

Rolf Menzel, Laboratory of Molecular Biology, National Institute of Diabetes, and Digestive and Kidney Diseases, National Institutes of Health, Bethesda, Maryland 20892.   *Present address:* Department of Research and Development, DuPont de Nemours, Wilmington, Delaware 19898.

Hillary C. M. Nelson, Department of Biology, Massachusetts Institute of Technology, Cambridge, Massachusetts 02139

Joanne M. Nickol, Laboratory of Molecular Biology, National Institute of Diabetes, and Digestive and Kidney Diseases, National Institutes of Health, Bethesda, Maryland 20892

Paul A. Overbeek, Laboratory of Molecular Genetics, National Institute of Child Health and Human Development, National Institutes of Health, Bethesda, Maryland 20892

Andrew Pakula, Department of Biology, Massachusetts Institute of Technology, Cambridge, Massachusetts 02139

Joram Piatigorsky, Laboratory of Molecular and Developmental Biology, National Eye Institute, National Institutes of Health, Bethesda, Maryland 20892

Dimitrina Pravtcheva, Department of Biology, Yale University, New Haven, Connecticut 06511

Mark Rabin, Department of Biology, Yale University, New Haven, Connecticut 06511

Donald C. Rio, Department of Biochemistry, University of California, Berkeley, California 94720

James M. Roberts, Department of Genetics, Fred Hutchinson Cancer Research Center, Seattle, Washington 98104

Gerald M. Rubin, Department of Biochemistry, University of California, Berkeley, California 94720

Frank H. Ruddle, Department of Biology, Yale University, New Haven, Connecticut 06511

Robert T. Sauer, Department of Biology, Massachusetts Institute of Technology, Cambridge, Massachusetts 02139

Azriel Schmidt, Laboratory of Molecular Biology, Division of Cancer Biology and Diagnosis, National Cancer Institute, National Institutes of Health, Bethesda, Maryland 20892

Marc J. Schulman, Department of Immunology, University of Toronto, Toronto, Ontario, Canada M5S 1A8

Philippe Soriano, Whitehead Institute for Biomedical Research, Massachusetts Institute of Technology, Cambridge, Massachusetts 02142

David Straus, Department of Bacteriology, University of Wisconsin, Madison, Wisconsin 53706

Robert Tjian, Department of Biochemistry, University of California, Berkeley, California 94720

William Walter, Department of Bacteriology, University of Wisconsin, Madison, Wisconsin 53706

Harold Weintraub, Department of Genetics, Fred Hutchinson Cancer Research Center, Seattle, Washington 98104

Robin A. Weiss, Institute of Cancer Research, Chester Beatty Laboratories, London SW3 6JB, England

Heiner Westphal, Laboratory of Molecular Genetics, National Institute of Child Health and Human Development, National Institutes of Health, Bethesda, Maryland 20892

Yan-Ning Zhou, Department of Bacteriology, University of Wisconsin, Madison, Wisconsin 53706

Contents

Chapter 4

√ *DNA Supercoiling as a Regulator of Bacterial Gene Expression*

   Martin Gellert and Rolf Menzel

Chapter 5

Retrotransposition in Yeast

   Gerald R. Fink

Chapter 6

Comparative Genetic Analysis of Homeobox Genes in Mouse and Man

   Frank H. Ruddle, Charles P. Hart, Mark Rabin,
   Anne Ferguson-Smith, and Dimitrina Pravtcheva

Chapter 7

Eukaryotic Transcriptional Specificity Conferred by DNA-Binding Proteins

James T. Kadonaga, Michael R. Briggs, and Robert Tjian

Chapter 8

Chromatin Structure Near an Expressed Gene

*Gary Felsenfeld, Beverly M. Emerson, P. David Jackson,
Catherine D. Lewis, Joanne E. Hesse, Michael R. Lieber,
and Joanne M. Nickol*

Chapter 12

Mapping and Manipulating Immunoglobulin Functions

Marc J. Shulman

Chapter 13

*T4: A T-Cell Surface Protein Mediating Cell–Cell and Cell–
AIDS Virus Interactions*

*Angus G. Dalgleish, Paul J. Maddon, Dan R. Littman,
Paul R. Clapham, Maurice Godfrey, Leonard Chess,
Robin A. Weiss, J. Steven McDougal, and Richard Axel*

Chapter 14

Identifying the Determinants of Protein Function and Stability

Robert T. Sauer, Hillary C. M. Nelson, Michael H. Hecht, and Andrew Pakula

The Role of Cis- and Trans-Acting Functions in Simian Virus 40 Gene Regulation

GEORGE KHOURY, KAMEL KHALILI,
JANET DUVALL, and JOHN BRADY

1. Introduction

Simian virus 40 (SV40) is a small DNA tumor virus, the circular genome [5243 base pairs (bp)] of which encodes at least two early proteins and four late gene products (Tooze, 1980). The lytic cycle of this virus is expressed over a temporal course in permissive African green monkey kidney cells. Early viral gene expression is predominant in the first 10–12 hr postinfection. The early viral program appears to be represented by a single transcription unit that gives rise to one primary messenger RNA (mRNA). This transcript is then differentially spliced into one of two mRNAs that encode the two early SV40 proteins, large tumor (large-T) and small tumor (small-t) antigens. All subsequent events in the lytic cycle appear to depend on the presence of a functional large-T antigen, which, through binding to three large-T-antigen-binding sites near the origin for DNA replication: (1) modulates downward the level of early gene transcription through a repressorlike function, (2) stimulates the initiation of viral DNA replication, and (3) both directly and indirectly activates the SV40 late transcriptional program (see Fig. 1). A set of late mRNA mole-

GEORGE KHOURY, KAMEL KHALILI, JANET DUVALL, and JOHN BRADY • Laboratory of Molecular Virology, National Cancer Institute, National Institutes of Health, Bethesda, Maryland 20892.

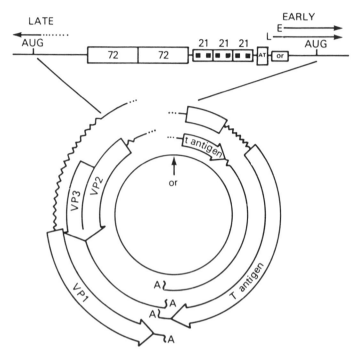

Figure 1. Genomic map and control region of SV40. The diagram presents the control region for expression of the SV40 early genes (large-T and small-t antigens) and late genes (VP1, 2, and 3). The origin for viral DNA replication (or) is flanked by the early transcriptional control sequences, including the Goldberg–Hogness box (AT), the three 21-bp repeats (each containing two copies of a GC-rich hexanucleotide), and the tandem 72-bp enhancer element. The early transcripts are initiated predominantly at position E early in infection and shift to position L after DNA replication. The late viral transcripts have heterogeneous 5′ ends, indicated by dots. Reprinted from Hamer and Khoury (1983) with permission.

cules encodes the structural proteins of SV40, namely, VP1, VP2, and VP3. In addition, a 61-amino-acid polypeptide, the agnoprotein, is made late in the lytic cycle. While the function of this protein is not entirely clear, it appears to play a role in encapsidation or assembly of the mature viral particles. Furthermore, the late agnoprotein may play a role in regulation of late gene expression.

For some time, SV40 and the other small DNA viruses have served as model systems for the elucidation of the *cis*-dependent control sequences as well as the *trans*-acting regulatory proteins that modulate expression of eukaryotic transcriptional units. We describe in the following sections a series of experiments directed at defining these *cis*- and *trans*-acting functions in the regulation of the SV40 early and late gene transcriptional programs.

2. Early Viral Transcriptional Program

Since SV40 enters the cell with no known viral enzymes, the earliest transcriptional events depend on the presence of cellular factors, including RNA polymerase II, that interact with the *cis*-dependent early viral transcriptional control signals. At least three upstream sequence elements have been defined that apparently associate with cellular factors to achieve efficient early virus gene expression (see Fig. 1). These include the Goldberg–Hogness or TATA box (adjacent to the origin of viral DNA replication) (Benoist and Chambon, 1981; Ghosh *et al.*, 1981); three 21-bp repeats, each containing the hexanucleotide GGGCGG (Fromm and Berg, 1982; Everett *et al.*, 1983; Hansen and Sharp, 1983; Baty *et al.*, 1984; Barrera-Saldana *et al.*, 1985; Dynan and Tjian, 1985); and the 72-bp tandem repeat that serves as an enhancer element increasing the efficiency of early viral transcription between 100- and 1000-fold (Banerji *et al.*, 1981; Gruss *et al.*, 1981; Moreau *et al.*, 1981).

As a classic enhancer element, the 72-bp repeat of SV40 functions in a relatively position- and orientation-independent fashion relative to the proximal promoter elements located immediately adjacent to the initiation site for transcription. Although the cellular factors that interact with the SV40 enhancer element have not yet been defined, a number of deletion and point mutations have identified nucleotide sequences within this repeat element that are critical for the functional activity of the enhancer (Weiher *et al.*, 1983; Zenke *et al.*, 1986). It appears clear at present that a single copy of the 72-bp element is sufficient for transcriptional enhancement, at least in tissue-culture systems. The selective advantage of two copies of this sequence, which has clearly been evolutionarily conserved, remains to be determined. Recent studies to demonstrate the dependence of *in vitro* transcription on the SV40 enhancer element have met with mixed success. Most notable among the positive results are those from Chambon's laboratory, which indicate that at least at the 5′ end of the transcription unit, the enhancer does appear to confer as much as a 10- to 15-fold stimulation of transcription using modified nuclear extracts (Sassone-Corsi *et al.*, 1984, 1985; Wildeman *et al.*, 1984).

The proximal promoter element, the TATA or Goldberg–Hogness box, has been shown *in vivo* to dictate the preferred 5′ ends of initiated transcripts. This element also contributes to the efficiency of transcription *in vivo* and *in vitro*. In the absence of the TATA box, transcription is still observed (Benoist and Chambon, 1981; Ghosh *et al.*, 1981), but the variability in the position of the 5′ ends of the transcripts increases.

The third, or central, transcription element identified as crucial for early SV40 gene expression is encompassed within the three 21-bp repeats in the form of six GC-rich hexanucleotides (see Fig. 1). This element has been shown by Tjian and his collaborators to interact with a cellular transcription factor, Sp1, that presumably contributes to the role of the element in transcription of the early SV40 template (see Dynan and Tjian, 1985). In the absence of the 21-bp repeats, both *in vivo* and *in vitro* transcription are substantially depressed. A similar element has been located within the transcriptional control sequences of a number of other viral and eukaryotic genes. At least the first (or proximal) three GC-rich boxes within the 21-bp repeats are critical to the activation of early transcription.

In a set of experiments described below, we attempted to define the role of these GC-rich repeats relative to the TATA box in terms of the initiation sites of efficient early viral transcription *in vivo* and *in vitro*. By analyzing transcription from a number of mutant templates containing insertions of increasing length between the TATA box and the 21-bp repeats, we demonstrated, first, that the TATA box functions efficiently only when immediately adjacent to the GC-rich sequences. Second, when sufficient space is interposed between these two early transcriptional control elements, the GC-rich sequences are predominant in dictating the preferred 5′ ends for initiation of transcription.

Studies of the potential interactions between transcriptionally important proteins associating with the TATA box and GC-rich sequences of SV40 employed either the wild-type virus or the mutants developed by Innis and Scott (1984), in which 4, 42, 90, or 130 nucleotides have been inserted between the Goldberg–Hogness sequence and the GC-rich hexanucleotides (see Fig. 2). In place of SV40 large-T antigen in the early-region coding sequences, we have inserted the bacterial gene that encodes chloramphenicol acetyl-transferase (CAT) (Gorman *et al.*, 1982). Thus, expression from these mutants can be easily assayed not only at the RNA level but also at the protein level. Furthermore, the elimination of large-

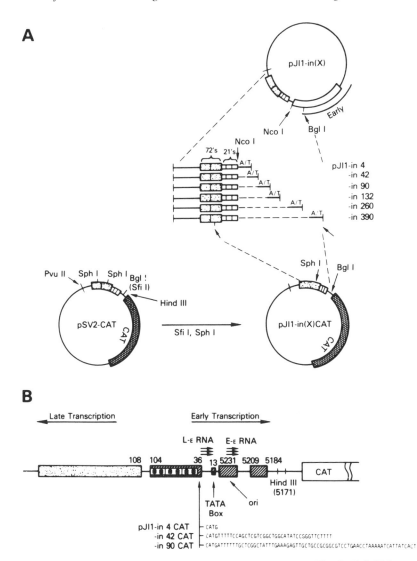

Figure 2. (A) Structure of the SV40 pJI1-in(X) CAT constructs. The *Bgl*I–*Sph*I fragment from insertion mutants (Innis and Scott, 1984) was ligated into the unique *Sfi*I–*Sph*I restriction sites in pSV2-CAT, yielding pJI1–CAT, pJI1–in4 CAT, pJI1–in42 CAT, and pJI1–in90 CAT. (B) Schematic diagram of the regulatory region of the SV40 early promoter in pJI1–in(X) CAT plasmids. The origin of replication, large-T-antigen-binding sites I, II, and III (hatched boxes), TATA box, GC-rich motifs (black boxes) within the 21-bp repeats, one copy of the 72-bp enhancer element (stippled box), and the 5' ends of E_E and L_E RNA are depicted. The nucleotide sequence contained in insertion mutations pJI1–in4, –in42, and –in90 CAT, as determined by Innis and Scott (1984), is presented below the schematic.

T antigen prevents autoregulation and DNA replication that would add considerable complexity to the analysis. Each of the mutants was introduced separately by DNA transfection in the presence of calcium phosphate into CV-1 monkey kidney cells, and the levels of RNA produced from equivalent amounts of DNA were assayed from the wild-type construct and each mutant by the S1 nuclease procedure. The results of a typical S1 profile are presented in Fig. 3.

It should be noted that under physiological conditions, wild-type SV40 produces two major species of early mRNA (Ghosh and Lebowitz, 1981; Wasylyk *et al.*, 1983; Buchman and Berg, 1984; Buchman *et al.*, 1984). Initially on infection, RNA is synthesized from the downstream initiation site near the origin for viral DNA replication. RNA originating from this initiation site is referred to as E_E RNA (see Fig. 2B). It is thought that large-T antigen, the early gene product, is produced, its binding to sequences near the origin for viral DNA replication sterically inhibits transcription initiation occuring at the E_E start site. A new set of upstream start sites, the late-early L_E start sites, then become functional (Fig. 2B). In the present study, substitution of the CAT gene for the large-T-antigen-coding sequences prevents the production of large-T antigen and thus eliminates this steric hindrance. As can be seen in Fig. 3 (lane 2), the wild-type construct generates a significant amount of E_E RNA. Insertion of 4 bp between the two early SV40 control elements leads to a significant reduction (5- to 10-fold) in the synthesis of E_E RNA and no concomitant use of other start sites (data not shown). As the insertion between the TATA box and 21-bp repeats increases to 42 or 90 nucleotides (Fig. 3, lanes 3 and 4), a complete shift in the site of transcriptional initiation occurs. Thus, in the absence of large-T antigen, a separation between these two early promoter sequences leads to a predominant use of upstream start sites. Two independent studies that also analyzed the effect of spacing between the SV40 early TATA box and upstream 21-bp repeats have reported similar findings (Barrera-Saldana *et al.*, 1985; Das and Salzman, 1985). It should be noted at this point that an identical shift in utilization of E_E or L_E RNA initiation sites can be duplicated in an *in vitro* transcription system with these insertion mutants using nuclear extracts from uninfected HeLa cells (data not shown). The most reasonable interpretation of the results would seem to be that the GC elements are a critical sequence in the control of initiation of early SV40 transcription. If the 21-bp repeats are adjacent to the TATA box, the latter sets the 5′

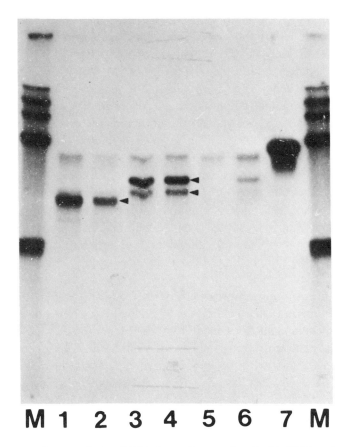

M 1 2 3 4 5 6 7 M

Figure 3. S1 nuclease analysis of RNA from cells transfected with SV40 early promoter insertion mutants. Transfection of CV-1 cells was performed by the calcium phosphate precipitation method. Each transfection mix contained 10 μg of the recombinant plasmid and 20 μg of carrier salmon sperm DNA. For the S1 probe, an *Eco*RI to *Sph*I (converted to *Bgl*II) fragment of DNA from pSV2-CAT was cloned into the M13mp19 vector. The DNA strand complementary to SV40 early RNA was synthesized in the presence of [^{32}P]-dCTP, restricted with *Hind*II, and heat denatured, and the single-strand probe was isolated following electrophoresis in a 6% acrylamide–urea gel. Hybridization of SV40 E$_E$ and L$_E$ RNA is expected to protect DNA fragments of approximately 320 or 360 bases, respectively. RNA extraction and hybridization, S1-nuclease digestion, and electrophoresis were performed as described previously (Brady and Khoury, 1985). Lanes: (M) ^{32}P-end-labeled SV40 *Hinf*I marker DNA; (1) pSV2-CAT; (2) pJI1–CAT; (3) pJI1–in42 CAT; (4) pJI1–in90 CAT; (5) pJI1–CAT Enh$^-$; (6) pJI1–in90 CAT Enh$^-$; (7) control S1 probe.

ends for initiation of RNA transcripts. When the TATA sequence is separated from the GC-rich hexanucleotides of the 21-bp repeats, however, it appears to be ineffective. In this case, the initiation sites may be dictated by sequences within the 21-bp repeats (Mishoe *et al.*, 1984).

We also looked at gene expression at the protein level in cells transfected by these mutants employing the CAT assay. CAT protein activity can be quantitatively assayed by the ability of the enzyme to convert [^{14}C]chloramphenicol to one of its acetylated forms. This assay is sensitive and reproducible. As shown in Fig. 4, a significant amount of CAT activity is generated when the wild-type SV40 construct is transfected into monkey kidney cells. An 8- to 10-fold lower level is seen when the 4-bp insertion mutant, pJI1–in4, is employed, which is roughly proportional to the reduction in RNA levels obtained with this mutant. An interesting and striking result is obtained with the larger insertion mutants (pJI1–in42 and pJI1–in90). Little or no CAT activity is observed, in contrast to the considerable levels of RNA produced by these mutants (see Fig. 3). An understanding of this observation comes from an examination of the nucleotide sequence surrounding the 5′ ends of the RNA molecules (see Fig. 5). The abundant RNA made from the E_E start site in the wild-type construct is efficiently translated into CAT protein. The upstream shift in the 5′ ends seen with the larger insertion mutants, however, generates RNA molecules that have one or two AUG initiator codons interposed between the 5′ end of the message and the iniator AUG for CAT enzyme translation. We analyzed the effect of the upstream AUGs on translation in a separate study, in which we assayed the translational efficiencies of E_E and L_E RNA transcripts *in vitro*. Consistent with data obtained *in vivo*, the results of these studies indicate that L_E RNAs are inefficient templates for translation of the downstream AUG used for translation of large-T antigen (Khalili *et al.*, 1987). Thus, although abundant RNAs are made from the L_E start sites in these insertion mutants, the L_E RNAs are, in general, poor translational templates for CAT protein.

These results not only demonstrate the importance of the spatial orientation between the two early SV40 promoter elements, but also give an insight into a translational regulation mechanism that temporally affects the production of early SV40 proteins (large-T and small-t antigens). It would appear that although early strand-specific SV40 RNA continues to be made late in the lytic cycle, the use of L_E start sites renders these transcripts inefficient templates for translation of the large-T antigen.

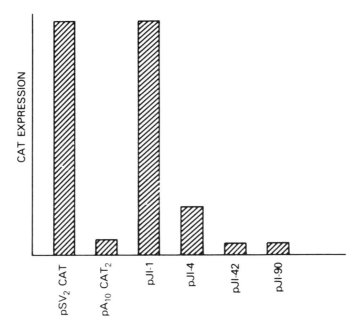

Figure 4. CAT activity in CV-1 cells transfected with pSV$_2$ CAT, pA$_{10}$ CAT$_2$, and pJI1-in(X) CAT constructs. Transfections were performed by the calcium phosphate precipitation method, containing 10 μg of each recombinant plasmid and 20 μg of carrier salmon sperm DNA. At 48 hr posttransfection, cell extracts were prepared and analyzed according to the protocol of Gorman *et al.* (1982). The percentage conversions (after correction for background) of chloramphenicol into its acetylated forms are pSV$_2$ CAT, 31%; pA$_{10}$ CAT$_2$, 0.7%; pJI-1, 32%; pJI-4, 4%; pJI-42, 0.2%; pJI-90, 0.4%. Reprinted from Loeken *et al.* (1986) with permission.

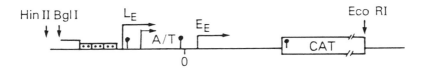

Figure 5. Diagram of the control region for expression of the CAT gene under the control of the SV40 early promoter. The positions of SV40 early-early (E$_E$) and late-early (L$_E$) RNAs are shown. The relative position of the CAT enzyme gene sequence is indicated in the open box. The positions of the CAT initiator AUG and two additional upstream SV40 AUGs that are present in L$_E$ RNA are shown by the lollipop symbol ( ).

3. Late Viral Transcriptional Program

Unlike the SV40 early regulatory unit, the SV40 late transcription unit functions inefficiently except late during the normal lytic cycle of the virus in monkey kidney cells. In nonpermissive cells, virus infection leads to a significant level of early gene expression, but transcription from the late promoter is weak or absent. These observations are of particular interest because the SV40 late transcription unit lacks some of the more common transcriptional control sequences of a typical polymerase II transcription unit. For instance, there is no well-defined TATA sequence upstream of the major late transcriptional initiation site. In addition, even though the SV40 early enhancer (72-bp repeat) works with either the early promoter or heterologous promoters in a manner that is relatively independent of orientation and position, this sequence is apparently unable to induce late transcription immediately after introduction of the gene into permissive or nonpermissive cells. In view of these unusual transcriptional properties, we have been interested in identifying mechanisms by which the late transcription unit is activated or positively regulated.

Recently, we and others have demonstrated that SV40 late gene expression can be activated by the SV40 early gene product, large-T antigen, even in the absence of DNA replication (Brady and Khoury, 1985; Brady *et al.*, 1985; Keller and Alwine, 1984, 1985). Induction of SV40 late gene expression has been obtained by either (1) cotransfection of a large-T-antigen-coding plasmid in *trans* with plasmid containing the late transcription unit or (2) introduction of the late transcription unit into COS-1 cells, an SV40-transformed CV-1 cell line that constitutively produces SV40 large-T antigen. S1-nuclease or Northern-blot analysis demonstrates that activation of the late transcription unit occurs at the level of RNA synthesis (Brady and Khoury, 1985). Since we routinely obtain more efficient *trans* activation in the COS-1 cell, the results presented below are obtained following introduction of the late transcription unit into this cell line. DNA replication was inhibited by the addition of cytosine arabinoside (30 μg/ml) to the culture media. Using a sensitive *Dpn*I replication assay, we have demonstrated that no amplification of the template occurs during the transient assay incubation period.

Studies in our laboratory using deletion and point mutants have defined two important domains for the SV40 large-T-antigen-induced late gene expression (Fig. 6) (Brady and Khoury, 1985). One of the regions important for *trans* activation includes large-T-antigen-binding sites I or

II or both. Deletion of large-T antigen-binding site I and one half of site II, as in mutant pSVs-L18, results in a late *trans*-activation induction level that is decreased to approximately 5–10% of that observed with the wild-type template (Fig. 6b). Similarly, deletion of 4 or 6 bp in large-T-antigen-binding site II dramatically reduces the efficiency of SV40 late gene expression (Fig. 6c and d). The other regulatory sequence required for efficient late gene activation is located in the SV40 72-bp repeats. Using a set of clustered point mutants that significantly affect early enhancer function (Weiher *et al.*, 1983) and are located in a single retained copy of the 72-bp repeats, we have found a parallel decrease in late gene expression (Fig. 6g–k); i.e., the sequences within the 72-bp repeats that serve as the SV40 early enhancer core element are apparently also important for late gene induction by large-T antigen in the absence of DNA replication. In contrast to the effect of mutations within the SV40 large-T-antigen-binding sites and the 72-bp repeats, mutations within the −25 region of the major late transcriptional initiation site that increase or decrease homology with the conserved eukaryotic TATA sequence did not affect the large-T-antigen-mediated *trans* activation of the late transcription unit (data not shown) (Brady *et al.*, 1985).

On the basis of these experiments, it was not possible to determine whether the transcriptional control sequences represent binding sites for *trans*-acting factors. To address this point, and to determine how the two upstream control elements interact to facilitate large-T-antigen-induced *trans* activation, we have used a template competition analysis (Brady and Khoury, 1985; Brady *et al.*, 1985). In the presence of a fixed amount of template and increasing levels of cloned competitor DNA fragments, which are capable of binding limiting *trans*-acting factors in the COS-1 cell, a decrease in SV40 late gene expression was observed. A typical competition assay, in which the entire SV40 late transcriptional regulatory sequence [SV40 map position (m.p.) 5171–272] has been used as the competitor DNA, is shown in Fig. 7. Standard transfection mixtures contained 0.1 μg of supercoiled SV40 template DNA plus a competitor DNA molecule cloned into plasmid pBR322. All competitor plasmids lacked the complete coding region for the major late gene product, VP1. Each competitor DNA plasmid was added at ratios of 1 : 1, 10 : 1, and 100 : 1 relative to the template DNA. Competition experiments in which the cloned DNA fragment contained three large-T-antigen-binding sites and the entire late promoter region (SV40 m.p. 5171–272) resulted in quantitative competition; the level of late gene expression was proportional to the ratio

Kpn I
(294) L$_{325}$

108   179   251

SV40 Late
Expression

Hind III   I   II   ↑   III   Pvu II   Hpa II
(5171)   (272)   (346)   BSC-1   COS-1
                    TATA
                    Box

		SV40	BSC-1	COS-1
a.	< ··· >	SV40	<1	100
b.	I ··· >	pSVs-L18	<1	5
c.	< ·········· I I ······················· > Δ6	SV40 6.1	<1	5
d.	< ·········· I I ·························· > Δ4	SV40 8.4	<1	5
e.	< ·· I I ······························· >	cs 1085	N.D.	N.D.
f.	< ················ I I ·············· >	SV40 dl 892	<1	100
g.	< ··············· I I ················ >	pSVTR 1	<1	100
h.	< ·· ·············· I xxxxx I ········· >	pSVTR 45	<1	100
i.	< ··············· I xxxxx Ixxl I ···· >	pSVTR 43	<1	30
j.	< ··············· I Ixxl Ixxl I ····· >	pSVTR 18	<1	15
k.	< ··· ············· I Ixxl Ixxl I ···· >	pSVTR 11	<1	10

Figure 6. SV40 late gene expression in COS-1 cells after transfection with template deletion and base-substitution mutants. Parallel cultures of BSC-1 and COS-1 cells were transfected with wild-type or mutant SV40 DNA templates (2 μg) by the calcium phosphate precipitation method. Mutant template pSVs-L18 contained SV40 sequences from map position (m.p.) 0 to 2754 cloned in a pBR322 derivative at the *Bam*HI site. Mutants SV40 6.1 and SV40 8.4 contained deletions of 6 and 4 bp, respectively, at the single *Bgl*I site of SV40. These plasmids contain the entire SV40 genome cloned into pMK16 at the *Bam*HI site. SV40 dl 892 contains a deletion of about 20 bp between SV40 m.p. 31 and 51. pSVTR 1, 45, 43, 18, and 11 are SV40 base-substitution mutants, described previously by Weiher *et al.* (1983). After transfection, cells were maintained in Dulbecco's Modified Eagle's Medium with fetal calf serum and cytosine arabinoside. At 40 hr posttransfection, whole-cell protein extracts were prepared, and 40-μl samples were analyzed by immunoblot analysis with anti-SV40 VP1 antiserum. The level of late gene expression was quantitated by excising the ^{125}I-band and determining the counts per minute in a gamma counter. The level of late gene expression observed from wild-type SV40 in COS-1 cells was arbitrarily set at 100%. (N.D.) Not determined. (■) GC-rich motifs; within the 21-bp repeats; (□) 72-bp repeats; (□) large-T-antigen-binding sites; (→) late transcription. Reprinted from Brady and Khoury (1985) with permission.

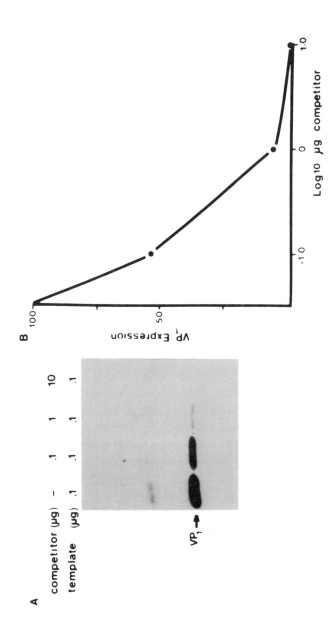

Figure 7. *In vivo* competition for *trans*-acting factor(s) present in COS-1 cells. COS-1 cells (10-cm plate) were transfected with template SV40 DNA and competing plasmid DNA by the calcium phosphate precipitation method. For the competition assays, standard transfection mixtures contained 0.1 μg of supercoiled SV40 template DNA plus a competitor DNA molecule containing the SV40 large-T-antigen-binding sites and late promoter (SV40 m.p. 517–272) cloned into pBR322 (see Fig. 6). All competitor plasmids lacked the complete coding region for the major late gene product VP1. Competitor plasmid DNA was added at a ratio of 1 : 1 (0.1 μg), 10 : 1 (1.0 μg), or 100 : 1 (10 μg) relative to template DNA. Transfected cultures were maintained in Dulbecco's Modified Eagle's Medium with fetal calf serum and cytosine arabinoside. At 40 hr posttransfection, whole-cell protein extracts were prepared and analyzed by immunoblot analysis with anti-SV40 VP1 antiserum (A), and the results were plotted (B). Reproduced from Brady and Khoury (1985) with permission.

of template to competitor DNA. For example, at a competitor template DNA ratio of 10 : 1, SV40 late gene expression was reduced to approximately 10% of that observed with no competitor DNA. The ability to compete for positive *trans*-acting transcription factors was dependent on the presence of SV40 control-region sequences, since no competition was observed with pBR322 or competitor plasmids containing certain fragments of the transcriptional control region (see below).

To locate more precisely the DNA sequences that were involved in binding the *trans*-acting factors present in COS-1 cells, the *in vivo* competition experiments were performed with a series of cloned DNA fragments containing deletions within the large-T-antigen-binding sites and the 72-bp repeats. We observed that deletion of either large-T-antigen-binding sites I and II (SV40 m.p. 5171–5243) or the 72-bp tandem repeats (SV40 m.p. 128–272) from the competitor plasmid resulted in markedly less efficient competition for the *trans*-acting factor (Brady *et al.*, 1985). In addition, neither of the control sequences alone was able to compete for the limiting *trans*-acting factor. These results suggested that efficient binding of the transcription factors required for SV40 late gene expression required the simultaneous interaction of one or more proteins with the two adjacent transcriptional control domains.

This hypothesis has been tested directly by analyzing the effect of an increase in the distance between two transcriptional domains on the efficiency of a particular competitor fragment (Brady *et al.*, 1985). A series of mutants (Innis and Scott, 1984) generated by the insertion of DNA sequences at the SV40 *Nco*I site (SV40 m.p. 37) were used as competitor fragments to test for binding of the limiting *trans*-acting factors. Insertion of 4 bp of DNA at the SV40 *Nco*I site had a minimal effect on the competition efficiency, reducing it by approximately 20%. In contrast, insertion of 42, 90, or 260 bp of DNA between the large-T-antigen-binding sites and the SV40 72-bp repeats resulted in inefficient competition by the competitor fragments with little or no decrease in the level of SV40 late gene expression. These results directly support the hypothesis that efficient binding of the *trans*-acting transcription factors requires a close physical relationship between the DNA sequences and therefore the putative transcription factors with which they bind.

4. Discussion

Although the sequences that control both SV40 early and late transcription are contained within a relatively short DNA segment (approximately 400 bp), the regulation of transcription is complex. Since SV40 has served in the past as a model for transcriptional regulation of eukaryotic genes, we can only assume at this point that other cellular transcription units will be at least as complex. The two major points that emerge from the results presented herein are discussed below.

First, our analyses of both SV40 early and late transcription suggest that efficient expression of these transcription units depends on the precise interaction of transcription factors that bind to independent, but adjacent, regulatory sequences. In the case of SV40 early gene expression, early-early (E_E) transcription requires a precise interaction between the TATA box and the adjacent upstream 21-bp repeats. Experiments from other laboratories have demonstrated that both these sequences correspond to DNA-binding sites for specific transcription factors. Davison *et al.* (1983) and Parker and Topol (1984) have described a TATA-box-binding protein. Similarly, Dynan and Tjian (1985 and references therein) have found that Sp1, a transcription factor isolated from uninfected HeLa cells, binds specifically to the SV40 21-bp repeats, making contact with the hexanucleotide sequences GGGCGG. Apparently, for SV40 early transcription, Sp1 must play an essential role in the stabilization of the TATA-box-binding protein and perhaps other transcription factors. This stabilization apparently requires more than a *cis* location, since the distance between the two binding sites is critical. When this interaction is disrupted, an alternative mode of transcription involving late-early (L_E) RNA initiation sites is activated. The sequences that control initiation from the L_E start sites have not been identified at this point, but the 21-bp would appear to be important. Thus, the 21-bp repeats, and presumably the transcription factor Sp1, are important factors not only in the efficiency of early transcription, but also as a major determinant of the selection of RNA initiation sites.

As with the regulation observed for the SV40 early transcription unit, *trans* activation of the SV40 late promoter by large-T antigen requires the interaction of transcription factors. We have previously shown that at least two upstream control regions are required for efficient induction of late transcription by large-T antigen (Brady and Khoury, 1985). The first sequence is located within large-T-antigen binding sites I and II. Although a direct role for large-T-antigen-binding in late gene activation has not been rigorously demonstrated, our results are consistent with such a mechanism (Brady *et al.*, 1984). The second critical sequence is located within the 72-bp repeats. It is of interest here that at least part of the sequences within the enhancer required for large-T-antigen induction are located with the enhancer core (Weiher *et al.*, 1983). Thus, although this sequence can efficiently induce transcription in the early direction, additional factors are apparently required to mediate late transcription. The similarities or differences in the 72-bp-repeat mediated activation of SV40 early and late transcription will become clear only when we have a molecular understanding of the mechanism that underlies transcriptional enhancement.

Our *in vivo* competition studies contribute additional information toward an understanding of the potential interaction of the transcriptional factors with the upstream sequences (Brady *et al.*, 1985). The ability to compete for transcriptional factors suggests a direct interaction of these factors with the adjacent late SV40 control sequences. For SV40 late transcription, efficient binding of the limiting transcription factors requires that the two control sequences be present in *cis* and at a critical distance from one another. These results suggest that efficient induction of late transcription requires an interaction between the proteins that bind to the independent regulatory sequences.

A similar conclusion regarding cooperative interaction of transcription factors was recently reported by Sawadogo and Roeder (1985) in their analysis of the binding proteins of transcription factors USF and TFIID to the adenovirus major late promoter. Dissociation-rate measurements suggested a cooperative interaction between USF and TFIID when simultaneously bound to the promoter DNA. Thus, the interaction of transcription factors may be a common mechanism for providing maximum transcriptional activity. It should be noted that the requirement of interaction for inducing RNA synthetic activity does not preclude a protein from binding to DNA by specific recognition, independent of other transcription factors. In fact, the available data from transcription factors such as Sp1, USF, and TFIID would support the concept of independent binding (Carthew *et al.*, 1985; Dynan and Tjian, 1985; Sawadago and Roeder, 1985).

A second important point elucidated by these studies concerns the quantitation of gene expression. Clearly, these experiments point out the potential problem in equating CAT activity with transcriptional activity. Since the CAT assay is widely used as rapid assay for the contribution of various promoters or enhancer elements to gene activity, one must first ascertain that there is good correlation between the level of RNA produced and the level of CAT enzyme synthesized for a given system.

ACKNOWLEDGMENT. We wish to express our gratitude to Marie Priest for the typing and preparation of this chapter.

References

Banerji, J., Rusconi, S., and Schaffner, W., 1981, Expression of a β-globin gene is enhanced by remote SV40 DNA sequences, *Cell* **27**:299–308.

Barrera-Saldana, H., Takahashi, K., Vigneron, M., Wildeman, A., Davidson, I., and Chambon, P., 1985, All six GC-motifs of the SV40 early upstream element contribute to promoter activity *in vivo* and *in vitro*, *Eur. Mol. Biol. Org. J.* **4**:3839–3849.

Baty, D., Barrera-Saldana, H. A., Everett, R. D., Vigneron, M., and Chambon, P. 1984, Mutational dissection of the 21-bp repeat region of the SV40 early promoter reveals that it contains overlapping elements of the early-early and late-early promoters, *Nucleic Acids Res.* **12**:915–932.

Benoist, C., and Chambon, P., 1981, *In vivo* sequence requirements of the SV40 early promoter region, *Nature (London)* **290**:304–310.

Brady, J., and Khoury, G., 1985, *Trans*-activation of the simian virus 40 late transcription unit by T-antigen, *Mol. Cell. Biol.* **5**:1391–1399.

Brady, J., Bolen, J. B., Radonovich, M., Salzman, N., and Khoury, G., 1984, Stimulation of simian virus 40 late gene expression by simian virus 40 tumor antigen, *Proc. Natl. Acad. Sci. U.S.A.* **81**:2040–2044.

Brady, J., Loeken, M. R., and Khoury, G., 1985, Interaction between two transcriptional control sequences required for Tumor-antigen-mediated simian virus 40 late gene expression, *Proc. Natl. Acad. Sci. U.S.A.* **82**:7299–7303.

Buchman, A. R., and Berg, P., 1984, Unusual regulation of simian virus 40 early-region transcription in genomes containing two origins of DNA replication, *Mol. Cell. Biol.* **4**:1915–1928.

Buchman, A. R., Fromm, M., and Berg, P., 1984, Complex regulation of SV40 early-region transcription from different overlapping promoters, *Mol. Cell. Biol.* **4**:1900–1914.

Carthew, R. W., Chodosh, L. A., and Sharp, P. A. 1985, An RNA polymerase II transcription factor binds to an upstream element in the adenovirus major late promoter, *Cell* **43**:439–448.

Das, G. C., and Salzman, N. P., 1985, Simian virus 40 early promoter mutations that affect promoter function and autoregulation by large-T-antigen, *J. Mol. Biol.* **182**:229–239.

Davison, B. L., Egly, J.-M., Mulvihill, E. R., and Chambon, P., 1983, Formation of stable preinitiation complexes between eukaryotic class B transcription factors and promoter sequences, *Nature (London)* **301**:680–686.

Dynan, W. S., and Tjian, R., 1985, Control of eukaryotic messenger RNA synthesis by sequence specific DNA-binding proteins, *Nature (London)* **316**:774–778.

Everett, R. D., Baty, D., and Chambon, P., 1983, The repeated GC-rich motifs upstream of the TATA box are important elements of the SV40 early promoter, *Nucleic Acids Res.* **11**:2447–2464.

Fromm, M., and Berg, P., 1982, Deletion mapping of DNA region required for SV40 early promoter function *in vivo, J. Mol. Appl. Genet.* **1**:457–481.

Ghosh, P. K., and Lebowitz, P., 1981, Simian virus 40 early mRNAs contain multiple 5′ termini upstream and downstream from a Hogness-Goldberg sequence: A shift in 5′ termini during the lytic cycle is mediated by T-antigen, *J. Virol.* **40**:224–240.

Ghosh, P. K., Lebowitz, P., Frisque, R. J., and Gluzman, Y., 1981, Identification of a promoter component involved in positioning the 5′ termini of simian virus 40 early mRNAs, *Proc. Natl. Acad. Sci. U.S.A.* **78**:100–104.

Gorman, C. M., Moffat, L. F., and Howard, B., 1982, Recombinant genomes which express chloramphenicol acetyltransferase in mammalian cells, *Mol. Cell. Biol.* **2**:1044–1051.

Gruss, P., Dhar, R., and Khoury, G., 1981, Simian virus 40 tandem repeated sequences as an element of the early promoter, *Proc. Natl. Acad. Sci U.S.A.* **78**:943–947.

Hamer, D. H., and Khoury, G., 1983, Introduction, in: *Enhancers and Eukaryotic Gene Expression* (Y. Gluzman and T. Shenk, eds.), Cold Spring Harbor Laboratory, Cold Spring Harbor, New York, pp. 1–15.

Hansen, U., and Sharp, P., 1983, Sequences controlling *in vitro* transcription of SV40 promoters, *Eur. Mol. Biol. Org. J.* **2**:2293–2303.

Innis, J., and Scott, W., 1984, DNA replication and chromatin structure of simian virus 40 insertion mutants, *Mol. Cell. Biol.* **4**:1499–1507.

Keller, J. M., and Alwine, J. C., 1984, Activation of the SV40 late promoter: Direct effects in the absence of DNA replication, *Cell* **36**:381–389.

Keller, J. M., and Alwine, J. C., 1985, Analysis of an activatable promoter: Sequences in the simian virus 40 late promoter required for T-antigen-mediated *trans* activation, *Mol. Cell. Biol.* **5**:1859–1869.

Khalili, K., Brady, J., and Khoury, G., 1987, Translational regulation of SV40 early mRNA defines a new viral protein, (submitted)

Loeken, M. R., Khalili, K., Khoury, G., and Brady, J., 1986, Evidence that polymerase II transcription requires interaction between proteins binding to control sequences, in: *Cancer Cells, Vol. 4: DNA Tumor Viruses. Control of Gene Expression and Replication* (M. Botcham, T. Grodticker, and P. Sharp, eds.), Cold Spring Harbor Laboratory, Cold Spring Harbor, New York (in press).

Mishoe, H., Brady, J. N., Radonovich, M., and Salzman, N. P., 1984, Simian virus 40 guanine–cytosine-rich sequences function as independent transcriptional control elements *in vitro*, *Mol. Cell. Biol.* **4**:2911–2920.

Moreau, P., Hen, R., Wasylyk, B., Everett, R., Gaub, M. P., and Chambon, P., 1981, The SV40 72 base pair repeat has a striking effect on gene expression both in SV40 and other chimeric recombinants, *Nucleic Acids Res.* **9**:6047–6068.

Parker, C. S., and Topol, J., 1984, A *Drosophila* RNA polymerase II transcription factor contains a promoter region specific DNA binding activity, *Cell* **36**:357–369.

Sassone-Corsi, P., Dougherty, J. P., Wasylyk, B., and Chambon, P., 1984, Stimulation of *in vitro* transcription from heterologous promoters by the simian virus 40 enhancer, *Proc. Natl. Acad. Sci. U.S.A.* **81**:308–312.

Sassone-Corsi, P., Wildeman, A., and Chambon, P., 1985, A *trans*-acting factor is responsible for the simian virus 40 enhancer activity *in vitro*, *Nature (London)* **313**:458–463.

Sawadogo, M., and Roeder, R. G., 1985, Interaction of a gene-specific transcription factor with the adenovirus major late promoter upstream of the TATA box region, *Cell* **43**:165–175.

Tooze, J. (ed.), 1981, *The Molecular Biology of Tumor Viruses*, 2nd ed., Part 2, Cold Spring Harbor Laboratory, Cold Spring Harbor, New York.

Wasylyk, B., Wasylyk, C., Matthes, H., Wintzerith, M., and Chambon, P., 1983, Transcription from the SV40 early-early and late-early overlapping promoters in the absence of DNA replication, *Eur. Mol. Biol. Org. J.* **2:**1605–1611.

Weiher, H., König, M., and Gruss, P., 1983, Multiple point mutations affecting the simian virus 40 enhancer, *Science* **219:**626–631.

Wildeman, A. G., Sassone-Crosi, P., Grundström, T., Zenke, M., and Chambon, P., 1984, Stimulation of *in vitro* transcription from the SV40 early promoter by the enhancer involves a specific *trans*-acting factor, *Eur. Mol. Biol. Org. J.* **3:**3129–3133.

Zenke, M., Grundström, T., Matthes, H., Wintzerith, M., Schatz, C., Wildeman, A., and Chambon, P., 1986, Multiple sequence motifs are involved in SV40 enhancer function, *Eur. Mol. Biol. Org. J.* **5:**387–397.

2

Regulation of the Heat-Shock Response in Escherichia coli

CAROL GROSS, DEBORAH COWING, JAMES ERICKSON,
ALAN GROSSMAN, DAVID STRAUS, WILLIAM WALTER,
and YAN-NING ZHOU

1. Introduction

Cells respond to a sudden increase in temperature by increasing their rate of synthesis of a small number of proteins (reviewed in Neidhardt *et al.*, 1984; Schlesinger *et al.*, 1982). This response is called the *heat-shock response*, and the proteins synthesized in response to heat stress are called the *heat-shock proteins* (HSPs). Both prokaryotes and eukaryotes have been shown to have a heat-shock response (Schlesinger *et al.*, 1982). At least two of the HSPs are strongly conserved between prokaryotes and eukaryotes (Bardwell and Craig, 1984), suggesting that the response serves a similar function in all organisms.

When *Escherichia coli* cells are shifted to a higher growth temperature, the rate of synthesis of the HSPs increases for about 10 min after temperature shift and then declines (shutoff) to a new steady-state rate of synthesis greater than the low-temperature rate. The amount of increase after temperature shift is characteristic for each protein. After a shift from 30 to 42°C, the increase in synthesis is 5- to 20-fold. The magnitude of the increase in HSP synthesis is greater after a shift to a higher tempera-

CAROL GROSS, DEBORAH COWING, JAMES ERICKSON, ALAN GROSSMAN, DAVID STRAUS, WILLIAM WALTER, *and* YAN-NING ZHOU • Department of Bacteriology, University of Wisconsin, Madison, Wisconsin 53706.

ture (Lemaux *et al.*, 1978; Neidhardt *et al.*, 1984). When cells are shifted to the lethal temperature of 50°C, most proteins synthesized are HSPs. In addition, at 50°C, the response is not transient. Production of HSPs continues as long as the cell is capable of making proteins (Fig. 1).

A total of 17 HSPs have been identified in *E. coli* (Neidhardt *et al.*, 1984). The function of most of these proteins is not clear. However, mutations that eliminate the heat response make the cell temperature-sensitive (Neidhardt and VanBogelen, 1981; Yamamori and Yura, 1982; Tobe *et*

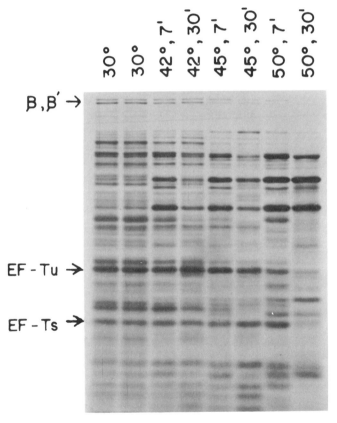

Figure 1. Heat-shock response at several temperatures. Strain SC122, growing exponentially at 30°C, was pulse-labeled with ^{35}S-methionine at 30°C or shifted to 42, 45, or 50°C and pulse-labeled with ^{35}S-methionine 7 or 30 min after shift to high temperature. Samples were taken into TCA and equal counts run on an SDS–polyacrylamide gel. Arrows on the right indicate HSPs.

al., 1984), indicating that the increased synthesis of at least some of these proteins after shift to high temperature is essential for growth.

We have been interested in determining how the production of the HSPs is controlled. In addition, we are investigating the function of the HSPs in *E. coli*. This chapter summarizes our studies in both these areas.

2. Transcription of the Heat-Shock Genes

The increased HSP synthesis after temperature upshift reflects increased transcription initiation from heat-shock gene promoters (Yamamori and Yura, 1980, 1982; Taylor *et al.*, 1984). Therefore, to understand the regulation of HSPs, it is necessary to identify heat-shock promoters and determine what is required for their transcription. We have mapped the promoters for four heat-shock genes (Taylor *et al.*, 1984; Cowing *et al.*, 1985) and have proposed a consensus sequence for these promoters (Cowing *et al.*, 1985). This consensus sequence differs from the consensus sequence for the majority of *E. coli* promoters (see Table I). We have purified the factor required for transcription of these promoters and find it to be a 32-kilodalton (kd) σ subunit (σ^{32}) of RNA polymerase (Grossman *et al.*, 1984). This factor is encoded by *rpoH (htpR)*, a gene known to be a positive regulator of the heat-shock response (Neidhardt and Van-Bogelen, 1981; Yamamori and Yura, 1982; Landick *et al.*, 1984; Yura *et al.*, 1984). Heat-shock promoters are recognized by RNA polymerase holoenzyme containing σ^{32} ($E\sigma^{32}$), while the predominant form of RNA polymerase holoenzyme ($E\sigma^{70}$) is not capable of initiating transcription from these promoters *in vitro* (Grossman *et al.*, 1984; Cowing *et al.*, 1985). The binding of $E\sigma^{32}$ at a heat-shock promoter protects the region surrounding the proposed consensus sequence from deoxyribonuclease (DNase) I digestion (Fig. 2).

The evidence suggests that the $E\sigma^{32}$ is responsible for most transcription from heat-shock promoters both before and after a temperature shift. The 5′ ends of the heat-shock gene transcripts made by $E\sigma^{32}$ *in vitro* are identical to the 5′ ends found for these transcripts *in vivo* at low temperature and after a heat shock, which is consistent with the idea that the same enzyme is carrying out transcription under both conditions (Cowing *et al.*, 1985). Mutations in *rpoH* eliminate the increase in transcription initiation from heat-shock promoters after a temperature shift (Yamamori and Yura, 1982; Cowing *et al.*, 1985; Taylor *et al.*, 1984). In strains con-

Table I. Sequences of Heat-Shock Promoters[a]

Promoter	−35 Region		−10 Region	+1
groE	TTTCCCCCTTGAA	GGGGCGAAGCCAT	CCCCATTCTCTGGTCAC	
dnaK P1	TCTCCCCCTTGAT	GACGTGGTTTACGA	CCCCATTTAGTAG TCAA	
dnaK P2	TTGGGCAGTTGAA	ACCAGACGTTTCG	CCCCTATTACAGACTCAC	
C62.5 gene P1	GCTCTCGCTTGAA	ATTATTCTCCCTTGT	CCCCATCTCTCCCACATC	
rpoD P$_{HS}$	TGCCACCCTTGAA	AAACTGTCGATGTGG	GACGATATAGCAG ATAA	
σ^{32} consensus	T tC CcCTTGAA	13-15 bp	CCCCATtTa	
σ^{70} consensus	TTGACA	16-18 bp	TATAAT	

[a]The sequences shown were determined as described in Cowing et al. (1985) and Taylor et al. (1984) and aligned as described in Cowing et al. (1985).

taining *rpoH165*, a poorly suppressed amber mutation, transcription from heat-shock promoters at 30°C is only 50% of that in wild-type (Cowing *et al.*, 1985; Goff *et al.*, 1984).

3. Regulation of rpoH and σ³²

The critical role of σ^{32} in transcription of the heat-shock genes indicates that understanding the regulation of σ^{32} is requisite to understanding how production of the HSPs is regulated. We have investigated both the transcriptional and the posttranscriptional regulation of σ^{32}. We find evidence that *E. coli* has several mechanisms for regulating σ^{32}, but we do not know how this regulation is related to the regulation of the heat-shock response. Our progress is summarized below.

We have determined the operon structure of the *rpoH* gene. S1 mapping of the 5′ and 3′ ends of *in vivo* messenger RNA (mRNA) shows that *rpoH* is the only gene in its transcriptional unit. The *rpoH* mRNA has four 5′ ends, located upstream of the start of the structural gene. The relative abundance of the 5′ ends is affected by temperature (see Fig. 3). There is one 3′ end, which had been predicted from the DNA sequence (Landick *et al.*, 1984). *In vitro* transcription shows that two of the 5′ ends correspond to transcripts initiated by Eσ^{70}. Eσ^{32} does not appear to transcribe *rpoH in vitro*. We do not know whether the other 5′ ends reflect processed mRNA or transcription initiations requiring additional regulatory factors. Preliminary experiments indicate that one of these mRNAs (mRNA-3) can be made in cell extracts under conditions in which none

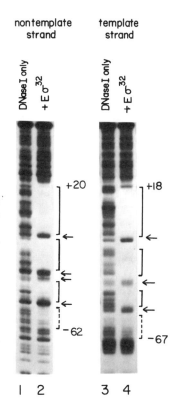

Figure 2. DNase I footprint of *rpoD* P$_{HS}$. DNA was labeled with ^{32}P upstream of *rpoD* P$_{HS}$, on either the template or the nontemplate strand. Samples (0.1 pmole) of DNA fragment were incubated with or without 2 pmoles Eσ^{32} for 10 min at 37°C. Poly(dAT) was added for 1 min to complete non-specific Eσ^{32}–DNA complexes. DNase I was then added for 30 sec. Lanes: (1) Nontemplate strand with DNase I; (2) nontemplate strand with Eσ^{32} and DNase I; (3) template strand with DNase I; (4) template strand with Eσ^{32} and DNase I. The extent of protection was determined by electrophoresis next to the same DNA fragment, subjected to Maxam–Gilbert sequencing reactions.

of the other mRNAs is synthesized. This implies that mRNA-3 is not a processed form, but results from a unique transcription initiation (J. Erickson, unpublished observations).

We have investigated what happens to the level of *rpoH* mRNA after temperature upshift. S1 mapping of both the 5′ and 3′ ends of *rpoH* mRNA indicates that it increases about 5-fold after a shift from 30 to 43.5°C (J. Erickson, unpublished observations). A similar result has been obtained with Northern blots (K. Tilly and C. Georgopoulos, personal communication). Although *rpoH* is not transcribed by Eσ^{32}, the kinetics of accumulation of *rpoH* mRNA follow those of the heat-shock response. Maximum accumulation occurs about 8 min after temperature shift (J. Erickson, unpublished data). We do not know whether the mRNA accumulation reflects increased synthesis or decreased degradation of the mRNA after temperature shift.

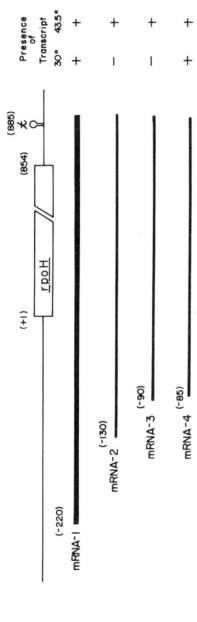

Figure 3. Structure of the *rpoH* transcription unit. The left portion of the figure diagrams the 5′ and 3′ ends of the *rpoH* mRNAs. The top line represents the DNA sequence with the location of the *rpoH* gene (+1 to 854) and the ρ independent terminator (*t*) shown. The numbers in the figure represent nucleotide positions relative to the *rpoH* initiation codon. The four species of *rpoH* mRNA (mRNA-1 through mRNA-4) are indicated below the DNA. The approximate position of the 5′ end of each mRNA is shown. All transcripts terminate at a series of Ts just downstream of the terminator (*t*). mRNA-1 and mRNA-4 originate from promoters recognized by Eσ[70]; the origin of the other mRNAs is unknown. The thickness of the lines represents the relative abundance of each mRNA at the time after shift to 43.5°C when the *rpoH* mRNA concentration is highest. The right section of the figure indicates the presence or absence of each mRNA at 30 and 43.5°C. (−) indicates that the mRNA is less than 5% of the total *rpoH* mRNA.

The rate of σ^{32} synthesis is also regulated posttranscriptionally, possibly by translational repression. We placed the *rpoH* gene under control of the λ P$_L$ promoter, regulated by the temperature-sensitive λ cI857 repressor. When λ repressor was inactivated by a temperature upshift, transcription from λ P$_L$ was turned on and σ^{32} was synthesized at a high rate. Within a short time, however, synthesis of σ^{32} declined about 10-fold from its peak rate. Control experiments indicate that production of galactokinase from the λ P$_L$ promoter in the same strain continued at a normal rate; thus, the shutoff of σ^{32} is not a result of decreased transcription initiation. Inhibition of σ^{32} synthesis is eliminated in a *dnaK* mutant.

One interpretation of these experiments is that the dnaK protein is a translational repressor of *rpoH* mRNA and that *dnaK* mutants are defective in translational repression. This would explain the already documented heat-shock phenotype of *dnaK* mutants, which are defective in the shutoff of the heat-shock response; after shift to high temperature, they continue to synthesize HSPs at a high rate (Tilly *et al.*, 1983). This phenotype could result from an inability of *dnaK* mutants to repress translation of the *rpoH* message. The continued high rate of synthesis of σ^{32} would prevent the normal shutoff of the heat-shock response.

Finally, we have found that σ^{32} is an unstable protein. When σ^{32} was overproduced from λ P$_L$ promoter following a shift from 30 to 42°C, its half-life was about 5 min (Fig. 4). Preliminary experiments suggest that σ^{32} stability decreases by a factor of 2 during the shutoff of the heat-shock response (D. Straus, unpublished data), indicating that altered proteolysis of σ^{32} may play a role in regulating the heat-shock response.

Our investigations suggest that *E. coli* can regulate the intracellular concentrations of σ^{32} in several ways, all of which may play a role in regulating the heat-shock response. It is known that the heat-shock response is induced by a variety of agents other than heat, including ethanol (Neidhardt *et al.*, 1984), infection with phage λ (Drahos and Hendrix, 1982; Kochan and Murialdo, 1982), DNA-damaging agents (Krueger and Walker, 1984), the stringent response (Grossman *et al.*, 1985), and unstable proteins (Goff and Goldberg, 1985). The inducers may act at different points to affect the regulation of σ^{32}.

4. Function of the Heat-Shock Proteins

Despite the evolutionary conservation of the HSPs, little is known about their function. We have been pursuing an observation we made

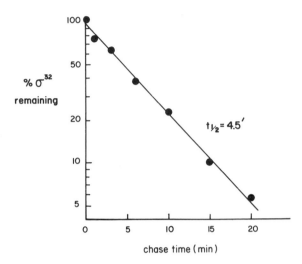

Figure 4. Instability of σ^{32} protein. Strain CAG 2059, which overproduces σ^{32} from the λ P$_L$ promoter (Grossman *et al.*, 1984), was grown at 30°C, shifted to 42°C, pulse-labeled with ^{3}H-leucine and ^{3}H-lysine from 5 to 8 min after shift, and chased with cold leucine and lysine. Samples were withdrawn beginning at 9 min ($t = 0$) after temperature shift and TCA-precipitated. ^{35}S-Methionine-labeled standard cells were added to samples prior to two-dimensional gel analysis to control for differential recovery (Gross *et al.*, 1984). Each point represents the ratio

$$\frac{(\text{dpm in } \sigma^{32} \text{ at time t})/(\text{dpm in } \sigma^{32} \text{ at time 0})}{(\text{dpm in total protein at time t})/(\text{dpm in total protein at time 0})}$$

several years ago that mutations in *rpoH* result in a defect in proteolysis as well as a defective heat-shock response (Baker *et al.*, 1984; Goff *et al.*, 1984). It has been suggested that altered proteolysis is important in recovering from a heat stress (Finley *et al.*, 1984; Goff *et al.*, 1984). One HSP, *lon* (Phillips *et al.*, 1984), is known to be involved in proteolysis (Gottesman and Zipser, 1978; Charette *et al.*, 1981; Chung and Goldberg, 1981). We have asked whether any of the other known mutations in HSPs alter proteolysis.

Mutations exist in *dnaK, dnaJ, groES, groEL,* and *grpE*, all of which prevent the growth of bacteriophage λ (reviewed in Neidhardt *et al.*, 1984). We have used two measures of the cellular capacity for proteolysis: the rate of degradation of the X90 fragment of β-galactosidase and the degradation of puromycyl fragment. The *lacZX90* mutation is a very late nonsense mutation in the *lacZ* gene that results in an unstable β-galactosidase fragment, X90 (Bukhari and Zipser, 1973). The degradation of X90 was originally used to measure the altered proteolysis phenotype of *lon* mutants (Bukhari and Zipser, 1973; Gottesman and Zipser, 1978). Puromycin causes premature termination of polypeptide chains, resulting in unstable polypeptides (Goldberg, 1972). Goldberg and his collaborators have used this assay as a measure of proteolysis (Goldberg, 1972; Goff *et al.*, 1984). Several years ago, Goff *et al.* (1984) demonstrated that an *rpoH* mutant was defective in degrading protein fragments generated by puromycin treatment.

The *dnaJ, grpE,* and *dnaK* mutations, as well as *lon* mutations, alter the degradation of X90 (Table II). The *dnaJ* mutant degrades X90 more slowly than wild-type at both 30 and 42°C. In *grpE* and *dnaK* mutants at 30°C, degradation of X90 is enhanced, while at 42°C, degradation of X90 is decreased.

The *dnaK, dnaJ, groES, groEL,* and *grpE* mutants are defective in the degradation of puromycyl fragments at both 30 and 42°C (Table II). The extent of the defect is equal to or greater than that in *lon* mutants (C. Gross, unpublished data). In future experiments, we will address the interrelationships among these proteins. We speculate that they may work as a complex in which mutation of any of the members results in a defect in proteolysis.

These data show that some of the HSPs affect proteolysis. Whether this effect is direct or indirect remains to be determined by *in vitro* experiments.

Table II. Proteolysis Phenotypes of Strains Carrying Mutations in Heat-Shock Genes

Strain	Degradation of β-gal X90[a]		Degradation of puromycyl fragments[a]	
	30°C	42°C	30°C	42°C
C600 X90/F' X90	+	+	+	+
lon::Tn10[b]	−	−	−	−
dnaK756[c]	+ +	−	−	−
grpE280[c]	+ +	−	−	−
dnaJ259[c]	−	−	−	−
groES30[c]	+	+	−	−
groEL140[c]	+	+	−	−

[a](−) Indicates that degradation is less than that shown by the wild-type; (+) indicates that degradation is equal to that shown by the wild-type; (+ +) indicates that degradation is greater than that shown by the wild-type.
[b]This mutation was obtained from S. Gottesman and transduced into the wild-type C600 X90/F' X90.
[c]These mutations were obtained from C. Georgopoulos and transduced into the wild-type C600 X90/F' X90.

5. Summary

The heat-shock proteins in *E. coli* are transiently overexpressed after shift to a higher growth temperature. The genes that encode the HSPs are preceded by promoters transcribed *in vitro* by a form of RNA polymerase holoenzyme containing a 32-kd σ subunit ($E\sigma^{32}$). The σ^{32} subunit is encoded by the *rpoH* (*htpR*) gene, previously identified as a positive effector of the heat-shock response. Our evidence suggests that $E\sigma^{32}$ is the enzyme that transcribes heat-shock genes at all temperatures. The level of σ^{32} may be regulated at several points: Accumulation of *rpoH* mRNA is affected by temperature shift, σ^{32} synthesis is regulated posttranscriptionally, and σ^{32} is an unstable molecule with a $t_{1/2}$ of 5 min. Many mutations in the HSPs are shown to have defects in proteolysis.

References

Baker, T. A., Grossman, A. D., and Gross, C. A., 1984, A gene regulating the heat shock response in *Escherichia coli* also affects proteolysis, *Proc. Natl. Acad. Sci. U.S.A.* **81:**6779–6783.

Bardwell, J. C. A., and Craig, E. A., 1984, Major heat shock gene of *Drosophila* and the *Escherichia coli* heat-inducible *dnaK* gene are homologous, *Proc. Natl. Acad. Sci. U.S.A.* **81:**848–852.

Bukhari, A. I., and Zipser, D., 1973, Mutants of *Escherichia coli* with a defect in the degradation of nonsense fragments, *Nature New Biol.* **243:**238–241.

Charette, M. F., Henderson, G. W., and Markovitz, A., 1981, ATP hydrolysis-dependent protease activity of the *lon (capR)* protein of *Escherichia coli* K12, *Proc. Natl. Acad. Sci. U.S.A.* **78:**4728–4732.

Chung, C. H., and Goldberg, A. L., 1981, The product of the *lon (capR)* gene in *Escherichia coli* is the ATP-dependent protease, protease La, *Proc. Natl. Acad. Sci. U.S.A.* **78:**4931–4935.

Cowing, D. W., Bardwell, J. C. A., Craig, E. A., Woolford, C., Hendrix, R. W., and Gross, C. A., 1985, Consensus sequence for *Escherichia coli* heat shock gene promoters, *Proc. Natl. Acad. Sci. U.S.A.* **82:**2679–2683.

Drahos, D. J., and Hendrix, R. W., 1982, Effect of bacteriophage lambda infection on the synthesis of *groE* protein and other *Escherichia coli* proteins, *J. Bacteriol.* **149:**1050–1063.

Finley, D., Ciechanover, A., and Varshavsky, A., 1984, Thermolability of ubiquitin-activating enzyme from the mammalian cell cycle mutant ts85, *Cell* **37:**43–55.

Goff, S. A., and Goldberg, A. L., 1985, Production of abnormal proteins in *E. coli* stimulates transcription of *lon* and other heat shock genes, *Cell* **41:**587–595.

Goff, S. A., Casson, L. P., and Goldberg, A. L., 1984, The heat shock regulatory gene, *htpR*, influences rates of protein degradation and expression of the *lon* gene in *Escherichia coli*, *Proc. Natl. Acad. Sci. U.S.A.* **81**:6647–6651.

Goldberg, A. L., 1972, Degradation of abnormal proteins in *Escherichia coli*, *Proc. Natl. Acad. Sci. U.S.A.* **69**:422–426.

Gottesman, S., and Zipser, D., 1978, Deg phenotype of *Escherichia coli lon* mutants, *J. Bacteriol.* **133**:844–851.

Gross, C. A., Grossman, A. D., Liebke, H., Walter, W., and Burgess, R. R., 1984, Effects of the mutant sigma allele *rpoD800* on the synthesis of specific macromolecular components of the *Escherichia coli* K-12 cell, *J. Mol. Biol.* **172**:283–300.

Grossman, A. D., Erickson, J. W., and Gross, C. A., 1984, The *htpR* gene product of *E. coli* is a sigma factor for heat shock promoters, *Cell* **38**:383–390.

Grossman, A. D., Taylor, W. E., Burton, Z. F., Burgess, R. R., and Gross, C. A., 1985, Stringent response in *Escherichia coli* induces expression of heat shock proteins, *J. Mol. Biol.* **186**:357–365.

Kochan, J., and Murialdo, H., 1982, Stimulation of *groE* synthesis in *Escherichia coli* by bacteriophage lambda infection, *J. Bacteriol.* **149**:1166–1170.

Krueger, J. H., and Walker, G., 1984, *groEL* and *dnaK* genes of *Escherichia coli* are induced by UV irradiation and nalidixic acid in an *htpR*[+]-dependent fashion, *Proc. Natl. Acad. Sci. U.S.A.* **81**:1499–1503.

Landick, R., Vaughn, V., Lau, E. T., VanBogelen, R. A., Erickson, J. W., and Neidhardt, F. C., 1984, Nucleotide sequence of the heat shock regulatory gene of *E. coli* suggests its protein product may be a transcription factor, *Cell* **38**:175–182.

Lemaux, P. G., Herendeen, S. L., Bloch, P. L., and Neidhardt, F. C., 1978, Transient rates of synthesis of individual polypeptides in *E. coli* following temperature shifts, *Cell* **13**:427–434.

Neidhardt, F. C., and VanBogelen, R. A., 1981, Positive regulatory gene for temperature-controlled proteins in *Escherichia coli*, *Biochem. Biophys. Res. Commun.* **100**:894–900.

Neidhardt, F. C., VanBogelen, R. A., and Vaughn, V., 1984, The genetics and regulation of heat shock proteins, *Annu. Rev. Genet.* **18**: 295–329.

Phillips, T. A., VanBogelen, R. A., and Neidhardt, F. C., 1984, *lon* gene product of *Escherichia coli* is a heat-shock protein, *J. Bacteriol.* **159**:283–287.

Schlesinger, M. J., Ashburner, M., and Tissieres, A. (eds.), 1982, *Heat Shock from Bacteria to Man*, Cold Spring Harbor Laboratory, Cold Spring Harbor, New York.

Taylor, W. E., Straus, D. B., Grossman, A. D., Burton, Z. F., Gross, C. A., and Burgess, R. R., 1984, Transcription from a heat-inducible promoter causes heat shock regulation of the sigma subunit of *E. coli* RNA polymerase, *Cell* **38**:371–381.

Tilly, K., McKittrick, N., Zylicz, M., and Georgopoulos, C., 1983, The *dnaK* protein modulates the heat-shock response of *Escherichia coli*, *Cell* **34**:641–646.

Tobe, T., Ito, K., and Yura, T., 1984, Isolation and physical mapping of temperature-sensitive mutants defective in heat-shock induction of proteins in *Escherichia coli*, *Mol. Gen. Genet.* **195**:10–16.

Yamamori, T., and Yura, T., 1980, Temperature-induced synthesis of specific proteins in *Escherichia coli:* Evidence for transcriptional control, *J. Bacteriol.* **142:**843–851.

Yamamori, T., and Yura, T., 1982, Genetic control of heat-shock protein synthesis and its bearing on growth and thermal resistance in *Escherichia coli* K12, *Proc. Natl. Acad. Sci. U.S.A.* **79:**860–864.

Yura, T., Tobe, T., Ito, K., and Osawa, T., 1984, Heat-shock regulatory gene *(htpR)* of *Escherichia coli* is required for growth at high temperature but is dispensable at low temperature, *Proc. Natl. Acad. Sci. U.S.A.* **81:**6803–6807.

3

Negative Control of DNA Replication Revealed in Composite Simian Virus 40– Bovine Papillomavirus Plasmids

JAMES M. ROBERTS and HAROLD WEINTRAUB

1. Overview

We have begun an analysis of DNA sequences that function in the control of DNA replication in eukaryotic cells. Bovine papillomavirus (BPV) replicates as an extrachromosomal nuclear plasmid, duplicating each viral genome in synchrony with the host-cell DNA once and only once per cell division. Simian virus 40 (SV40) replication, however, is unresponsive to cellular controls, so the viral DNA replicates exponentially within the host-cell nucleus. To approach our study of the mechanisms of replication control, we designed a model system consisting of SV40 and BPV DNA sequences linked to create a hybrid replicon. We have obtained evidence that a main feature of copy-number regulation in the composite SV40–BPV plasmid is the imposition of dominant negative control encoded by BPV, which overrides the runaway replication induced by the positive factor, SV40 large tumor (large–T) antigen. Using a transient replication assay, we have previously been able to define the elements in the BPV genome that are sufficient to establish controlled replication in composite SV40–BPV plasmids (Roberts and Weintraub, 1986). These elements consist of two *cis*-acting sequences that are closely linked to BPV replication origins and a third element that acts in *trans*. The latter is en-

JAMES M. ROBERTS and HAROLD WEINTRAUB • Department of Genetics, Fred Hutchinson Cancer Research Center, Seattle, Washington 98104.

coded within the 5′ part of the E1 open reading frame (ORF) of the BPV genome and is physically and functionally separable from the positive replication factor encoded within the 3′ part of the same ORF. The controlled replication of SV40–BPV composite plasmids has enabled us to create permanent COS cell lines that stably maintain these plasmids as episomes.

2. Introduction

Eukaryotic chromosomes are organized into multiple replication units, and there are approximately 10,000 of these units per vertebrate genome (reviewed in Hand, 1978; see also Blumenthal *et al.*, 1973). Despite this complexity, there is the absolute requirement not only that each DNA sequence must be replicated once within each cell cycle, but also that it must be replicated *only* once. There must be a mechanism that prevents the reinitiation of replication on DNA that has previously been replicated.

One experimental approach to understanding the mechanisms of eukaryotic replication control involves studying relatively simple extrachromosomal elements that display replicative properties identical to those of the host-cell genome. BPV replicates as an extrachromosomal nuclear plasmid in rodent cells, stably maintaining a copy number of 100–200 moles per cell (Lancaster, 1981; Law *et al.*, 1981). Density-shift experiments have demonstrated that every BPV plasmid replicates, in parallel with the host-cell genome, just once per cell cycle (J. Reynolds and M. Botchan, unpublished data). Thus, BPV exhibits a regulated mode of DNA replication.

Both *cis-* and *trans*-acting elements within the BPV genome are necessary for BPV replication. Two complementation groups, encoding *trans*-acting factors that modulate BPV replication, have been identified. Viral mutants within the 3′ part of the E1 ORF fail to replicate, but can be complemented in *trans* by wild-type virus (Sarver *et al.*, 1984; Lusky and Botchan, 1985). Thus, the polypeptide encoded within the 3′ part of E1 is thought to be necessary for normal viral replication. Viral mutants in the E6 and E7 ORFs accumulate to only 1–2 copies per cell (Lusky and Botchan, 1985). The role of the E6/E7 gene product in viral replication is unclear; however, data indicate that it may function to enhance the level or activity of the E1 gene product (Berg *et al.*, 1986).

Electron microscopy of BPV replication intermediates demonstrates that replication eyes center at a discrete site within the BPV genome (Waldeck *et al.*, 1984). This is thought to be the replication origin. Consistent with this interpretation is the observation that plasmids containing this region of the BPV genome will replicate autonomously in cells harboring a wild-type BPV genome (which provides *trans*-acting replication factors). This site has been termed plasmid maintenance sequence I (PMS I) (Lusky and Botchan, 1984). Analysis of mutations within PMS I has identified a 117-base-pair (bp) region that is essential for PMS function (Lusky and Botchan, 1986).

PMS function also requires a linked enhancer sequence. A second site with PMS activity, PMS II, has been located within the E1 ORF (Lusky and Botchan, 1984). This site shows extensive sequence homology with PMS I and can support replication in viral genomes that contain mutations in PMS I; however, replication eyes have not been observed over this site (Waldeck *et al.*, 1984).

In contrast to BPV, lytic viruses such as SV40 escape cellular factors that control DNA replication. SV40 demonstrates a replication pattern that is uncoupled from the host cell's regulatory mechanisms so that each viral genome replicates multiple times within each cell cycle, ultimately killing the host cell (Roman and Dulbecco, 1975). The only viral information necessary for SV40 replication is the replication origin and the viral-encoded, *trans*-acting of large-T antigen (Tegtmeyer, 1972; Tjian, 1978; Meyers and Tjian, 1980). The escape of SV40 from the cellular copy-number-control system could be due to the absence of *cis*-acting sequences that can be recognized by the cell or to the intrinsic properties large-T-antigen-driven replication, which may override cellular controls.

We have begun an analysis of the BPV DNA sequences that function in the regulation of DNA replication (see Roberts and Weintraub, 1986). We initially approached this problem by designing experiments to examine whether the copy-number control exhibited by BPV is dominant or recessive to the runaway replication observed for SV40. To this end, we studied the replicative properties of hybrid molecules containing SV40 and BPV DNA sequences (see also DuBridge *et al.*, 1985). We found that in the presence of BPV-encoded *trans*-acting factor(s), BPV *cis*-acting sequences suppress runaway replication from the SV40 replication origin present on the same plasmid. Two BPV-encoded *cis*-acting sequences are necessary for replication control; these sequences are termed *negative control of replication* (NCOR) I and II: NCOR I is located within PMS I, while NCOR II is closely linked to PMS II. A *trans*-acting product encoded within the 5′ part of the E1 ORF is also required for replication control; however, this factor is distinct from the positively acting E1 gene product that maps to the 3′ part of the E1 ORF and that is necessary for DNA replication (Sarver *et al.*, 1984).

Because the PBV controlling elements can suppress the activity of the SV40 origin despite the presence of an excess of SV40 large-T antigen, these experiment suggest that regulation of DNA replication in eukaryotic cells may involve a negative control mechanism that can discriminate between replicated and unreplicated templates. Given these findings, we think that certain aspects of copy-number control in this system are mediated by a mechanism fundamentally different from the ones that have been demonstrated for prokaryotic plasmids. We show herein that in stable transformation assays, negative control by BPV is dominant over the runaway replication encoded by SV40.

3. Results

3.1. Construction of Composite Simian Virus 40–Bovine Papillomavirus Replicons

All the information necessary for regulated BPV replication is contained within a 5.4-kilobase (kb) *Hind*III–*Bam*HI fragment of the BPV genome (Lowy *et al.*, 1980; Law *et al.*, 1981; Sarver *et al.*, 1982; DiMaio *et al.*, 1982). This information includes the BPV replication origin (Waldeck *et al.*, 1984; Lusky and Botchan, 1984), three known transcriptional promoters (Heilman *et al.*, 1982; Sarver *et al.*, 1984; Stenlund *et al.*, 1985; M. Botchan, personal communication), at least two enhancers (Lusky *et al.*, 1983; Spalholz *et al.*, 1985), and eight ORFs (Chen *et al.*, 1982), three of which encode proteins that have been demonstrated to modulate BPV replication (Sarver *et al.*, 1984); Lusky and Botchan, 1985). The composite replicon pSV–BPV (Fig. 1) was constructed by joining this 5.4-kb subgenomic BPV fragment to the SV40 replication origin, which is contained within a 550-bp *Hind*III–*Hpa*I region of the SV40 genome. This fragment also contains the SV40 enhancer and the early and late promoters. The early promoter is positioned to transcribe the BPV sequences, ensuring a high level of expression of BPV gene products. A control construct, pSV (Fig. 1), includes no BPV sequences; it contains just the SV40 replication origin present in the *Hind*III–*Hpa*I 550-bp fragment. Replication from the SV40 origin requires an SV40-encoded protein, large-T antigen. The experiments described below utilize COS-7 cells, which provide SV40 large-T antigen in *trans* from cellular genomic copies of the SV40 large-T antigen gene (Gluzman, 1981).

3.2. Construction of Permanent Cell Lines Containing Simian Virus 40–Bovine Papillomavirus Composite Plasmids

Previous transient replication assays have shown that in some cases, composite SV–BPV plasmids exhibit regulated replication—they do not increase in copy number relative to the host-cell genome (Roberts and Weintraub, 1986). In contrast, the plasmid pSV exhibits unregulated "runaway" replication, increasing in copy number to more than 10,000 moles per cell by 72 hr posttransfection. Ultimately, pSV disappears from the transfected cell population as the runaway plasmid replication kills the host cell. These observations led us to predict that the isolation of permanent COS cell lines containing stably replicating SV40 origin plasmids should be facilitated by the linkage of the SV40 origin to BPV DNA sequences. To test this prediction, we compared the ability of the plasmid

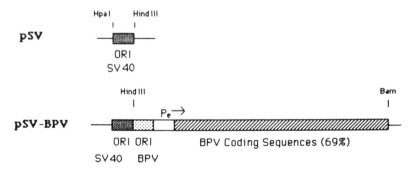

Figure 1. Construction of the pSV–BPV replicon. As described in the text, the plasmid pSV contains the SV40 replication origin, and the plasmid pSV–BPV contains the SV40 origin linked to a *Hind*III–*Bam*HI 5.4-kb subgenomic fragment of BPV that contains all the information necessary for regulated BPV replication. The cloning vector in both cases is pAT153, a "poisonless" derivative of pBR322.

pSV-Neo and the composite plasmid pSV-Neo–BPV to produce G-418-resistant cell lines on transfection into COS cells. Both plasmids contain the SV40 origin-promoter region that drives expression of the bacterial neomycin-resistance gene (Jimenez and Davies, 1980; Colbere-Garapin *et al.*, 1981; Southern and Berg, 1982). In addition, pSV-Neo–BPV contains the 5.4-kb *Hind*III–*Bam*HI BPV DNA fragment described above. We also compared the transfection efficiency of both constructs with that of the nonreplicating plasmid pRous-Neo. The pRous-Neo plasmid contains the Rous sarcoma virus long terminal repeat, which promotes expression of the *Neo^r* gene. It produces G-418-resistant colonies by integrating into the host genome and replicating under the control of adjacent host sequences.

We agree with previous observations (Tsui *et al.*, 1982) that the isolation of stable, drug-resistant colonies following transfection of COS cells with an SV40-origin-containing plasmid is a very rare event. After 2 weeks of selection in 0.5 mg/ml G-418 following transfection of COS cells with pSV-Neo, we observed predominantly small, slowly growing colonies of 10–20 cells (Fig. 2A). These abortive colonies are not observed in mock-transfected cell cultures and presumably represent the transient drug resistance afforded by pSV-Neo until its overreplication kills the host cells. In contrast, cultures transfected with pSV-Neo–BPV show an equivalent number of colonies, but these are robust and grow rapidly (Fig. 2A). The drug-resistant colonies observed following transfection with pSV-Neo–BPV are of equal size and about twice as abundant as those observed following transfection with an equimolar amount of pRous-Neo (Fig. 2A).

At 3 weeks of G-418 selection (Fig. 2B), the small colonies seen in the pSV-Neo transfection have died. A small number of large, actively growing colonies persist. Most of these colonies have proven difficult to subclone. However, we have succeeded in isolating a few stable G-418-resistant cell lines from pSV-Neo transfection and are currently investigating the state of the transfected plasmid in these cells. Unlike the drug-resistant colonies observed in the pSV-Neo transfection, the drug-resistant colonies obtained with the pSV-Neo–BPV plasmid all continue to grow at rates comparable to those obtained with the control plasmid pRous-Neo. In two independent experiments, 8- to 10-fold more stably growing G-418-resistant colonies were found 3 weeks posttransfection with pSV-Neo–BPV than with an equimolar amount of pSV-Neo.

To investigate the state of the plasmid DNA in these cells, we prepared total cellular DNA from a pool of about 100 independent G-418-

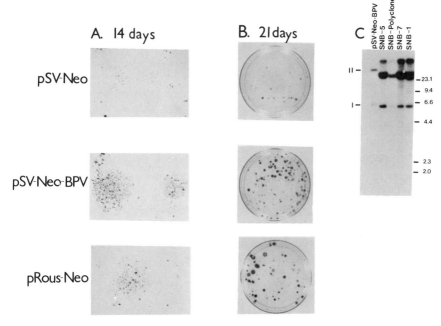

Figure 2. Construction of permanent COS cell lines with a pSV–BPV plasmid containing a selectable marker. Colonies of 5×10^5 COS-7 cells/plate were transfected with either 200 ng pSV-Neo, 200 mg pRous-Neo, or 300 ng pSV-Neo–BPV (equimolar amounts), and cells were selected for resistance to 0.5 mg/ml G-418. (A) Typical colonies obtained with each plasmid at 14 days posttransfection and continuous G-418 selection. (B) Stained plate of cells transfected with each plasmid after 21 days of selection in G-418. (C) Southern blot of 0.5 μg of uncut total cellular DNA isolated from a pool of about 100 colonies (SNB-polyclone) and from three independent clones (SNB-1, SNB-5, SNB-7) of G-418-resistant COS cell lines obtained following transfection with pSV-Neo–BPV. Also shown is a marker lane containing 100 pg of the uncut plasmid pSV-Neo-BPV; forms I and II are indicated. The probe is [^{32}P]-pSV-Neo–BPV.

resistant colonies obtained from the pSV-Neo–BPV transfection, as well as from several individual clones. In all cases, we found that pSV-Neo–BPV persists as a stable extrachromosomal plasmid at an average copy number of about 100–200 per cell (Fig. 2C). We have found the copy number of the pSV-Neo–BPV episome to be constant for at least 2 months of cell culture under continuous G-418 selection. We do not yet know whether the distribution of the plasmid is uniform among the cells in this population. Plasmid DNA that comigrates with genomic DNA is also observed in the Southern blot shown in Fig. 2C. The high-molecular-weight form of the transfected plasmid is approximately 5-fold more abundant than free supercoiled monomers, bringing the total copy number of pSV-Neo–BPV in these cells to about 500–1000 moles per cell.

We have considered the possibility that in the course of isolating G-418-resistant transformants, we may have selected for COS cell variants that stably maintain the pSV-Neo–BPV plasmid by virtue of diminished SV40 large-T-antigen synthesis. In principle, low large-T antigen levels could produce a cellular environment in which the copy number of an SV40 origin plasmid would be limited by the amount of available large-T antigen, thus effectively suppressing the lethal consequences of runaway plasmid replication. We considered this possibility unlikely for a number of reasons, including its failure to explain the difference in transfection efficiencies between pSV-Neo and pSV-Neo–BPV. Nevertheless, we used immunofluorescence to demonstrate that all the G-418 transformants we have isolated continue to synthesize as much large-T antigen as the parental COS cell population.

Consistent with this observation, we find that supertransfection of these cells with the plasmid pSV results in the amplification of the exogenous pSV plasmid, while the endogenous plasmid pSV-Neo–BPV maintains a stable copy number. However, amplication of the exogenous pSV DNA shows that it is only about one tenth the level of that in normal COS-7 cells. It seems likely that the endogenous copies of pSV-Neo–BPV have sequestered much of the functional nuclear large-T antigen, so that it is only partially available to drive replication of the supertransfected pSV plasmid. If this can be verified by direct measurement, it would suggest that the endogenous pSV-Neo–BPV plasmid replicates under copy-number control while harboring bound large-T antigen molecules, implying that the BPV exerts control on SV40 replication at a point subsequent to large-T-antigen binding. Consistent with the interpretation that large-T antigen has been sequestered by the endogenous plasmids is our observation that if additional large-T antigen is supplied to the system (as a large-T antigen gene on the supertransfected plasmid), then pSV amplifies to more normal levels (data not shown). Moreover, in a variant line that has lost over 70% of the pSV-Neo–BPV genomes, supertransfection with pSV yields levels of amplifications that are significantly higher and are similar to those seen in COS-7 cells.

The major conclusion we draw from these experiments is that the replication suppression of composite SV–BPV plasmids in transient replication assays is manifested in long-term transfection experiments in a manner similar to that in which the stable, controlled replication of SV–BPV plasmids is manifested in permanent COS cell lines. The stable maintenance of SV–BPV plasmids in COS cells does not directly suggest a mechanism by which this stable copy number is achieved. Copy-number control for BPV itself is accomplished through a mechanism that ensures that each viral genome replicates just once per cell cycle, implying that BPV is replicating under the host control system. We have recently performed density-shift experiments that indicate that the same mechanism may operate for the SV–BPV plasmids. These experiments show that both the integrated and episomal SV–BPV in stable cell lines also replicate just once per cell generation in coordination with the COS cell genome.

4. Discussion

4.1. Negative Control of DNA Replication

Eukaryotic genomes are all organized into multiple replication units. Mammalian genomes, for example, probably initiate DNA replication at over 10,000 sites during each cell-division cycle (see Hand, 1978). Replication does not begin simultaneously throughout the genome; instead, large numbers of replication-initiation sites are used in a sequential fashion. This temporal ordering of DNA replication means that the cell is constantly faced with the problem of distinguishing between replicated and unreplicated DNA. Regions of the genome that replicate early in S phase must not be rereplicated, since DNA synthesis is subsequently initiated at other places late in S phase.

We have used BPV as a model system to begin to analyze the molecular mechanism of replication control in eukaryotic cells. Linkage of BPV DNA sequences to the SV40 replication origin creates a composite SV–BPV replicon that exhibits controlled replication. In an environment in which large-T antigen, a *trans*-acting positive replication-initiation factor, is present in excess, the BPV genome can provide *cis*-acting, dominant signals that negatively control DNA replication. This interpretation is consistent with earlier observations concerning the control of cellular

DNA replication (Rao and Johnson, 1970). Those experiments demonstrated that fusion of G_1-phase cells to S-phase cells will induce DNA synthesis in the G_1 nucleus, suggesting that the onset of DNA replication in G_1 cells is limited by the availability of a diffusible, *trans*-acting positive factor present in the S-phase cell. However, fusion of G_2-phase cells to S-phase cells would *not* induce reduplication of the G_2 genome despite continued DNA synthesis in the companion S-phase nucleus, suggesting that the G_2 genome contains *cis*-dominant information that negatively regulates DNA replication.

Our main conclusion, therefore, is that in contrast to many bacterial mechanisms that seem to control the initiation of DNA synthesis by limiting the availability of initiator proteins or RNA, the SV–BPV chimera, and perhaps the cellular genome, is controlled by negative elements that override the functional interaction between positive initiator elements (e.g., SV40 large-T antigen) and the replication origin. Presumably, SV40 is a runaway replicon because it does not contain *cis*-acting sequences, which allow the host controlling factors functional and perhaps physical access to the SV40 genome.

In identifying the components of the BPV genome involved in replication control, we have relied on a transient replication assay that evaluates the replication kinetics of experimental and control plasmids over 48 hr (Roberts and Weintraub, 1986). Since a variety of DNA sequences have been observed to inhibit replication of SV40-origin plasmids (Lusky and Botchan, 1981; DeLucia *et al.*, 1986), one may question the extent to which our observations with SV–BPV composite plasmids reveal replication control rather than a nonspecific diminution in replication rate. We believe, for the following four reasons, that the replication suppression of SV–BPV plasmids represents replication control: (1) Suppression of replication requires *two* specific *cis*-acting elements. The presence of either element alone has no discernible effect on plasmid replication. (2) The suppressive effect of the two NCOR sites requires a specific BPV-encoded *trans*-acting factor. In the absence of this gene product, plasmids containing the two NCOR sites replicate equivalently to an SV40 control. (3) The three regulatory elements we describe have each been previously associated with BPV replicative functions using very different assays. The *trans*-acting factor is encoded within the E1 ORF. This has been shown to be a complex locus, the 5′ part being involved in the negative control of replication (Berg *et al.*, 1986) and the 3′ region providing a positive element for replication (Lusky and Botchan, 1985; Berg *et al.*, 1986). The two *cis*-acting NCOR sites are closely linked to, or overlap, BPV replication origins (Lusky and Botchan, 1984). (4) SV–BPV plasmids containing a selectable marker can be used to create permanent COS cell lines that stably replicate the composite plasmid as an episome. Thus, the replication suppression observed for 48 hr in a transient assay can extend indefinitely. Significantly, density-shift experiments demonstrate that the SV–BPV composite plasmids in the stable cell lines replicate once per cell cycle in concert with the host-cell genome, suggesting that these plasmids are replicating under the host-cell copy-number-control system. This observation could be used to identify cellular elements that impose copy-number control on SV40–Neo^r plasmids. Moreover, the availability of an *in vitro* replication system for SV40 should make it possible to re-create this type of control *in vitro* (Ariga and Sugano, 1983; Li and Kelly, 1984).

4.2. Mechanisms of Replication Control

Since BPV normally replicates in synchrony with the host genome, we assume that BPV is capable of reading and responding to those host factors that ensure that each host replicon initiates just once per cell cycle. Hence, it is likely that information about the means by which BPV controls its replication will reveal features of the means by which the cell controls its replication.

Since the NCOR sequences map so closely to known BPV origins, it is possible that negative control could be mediated during the process of initiating from the BPV origin. This is supported by the finding that an insertion mutation that inhibits BPV replication also inhibits negative control over SV40. However, we think that this hypothesis is not correct in its simplest form, since our attempts to show that the BPV origins are fully functional in these nonpermissive cells have indicated that they are not. For SV–BPV, therefore, negative control of reinitiation can be mechanistically separated from replication initiated at the BPV origin. Nevertheless, the origin and the sequences for negative control overlap for the normal BPV virus. It would be surprising if the two processes were not coupled. One possibility is that their proximity assures rapid inhibition immediately after a cell-cycle-controlled initiation event.

There is a major problem with trying to relate these "principles" of the negative control of replication of the composite SV–BPV replicon to the mechanism by which the cell might control DNA replication. The cellular genome consists of multiple replicons. As with BPV, we would guess that reinitiation for a given replicon might be inhibited by the binding of a negative, *trans*-acting host element to the host equivalent of two NCOR sites, possibly located near an origin. This explanation leaves an unanswered question, however: What determines that the negative element will bind to the recently replicated NCOR sequences and not to the NCOR sequences from an adjacent replicon that has not replicated? One possibility is that recognition takes advantage of the peculiar DNA structure (e.g., single-stranded regions or Okazaki fragments) of the replication fork itself. Other potential signals that might be unique to newly replicated DNA include transient hemimethylation of NCOR sequences or altered torsional stress associated with passage of the replication fork. The observation that newly replicated DNA is very rapidly methylated (Koshet *et al.*, 1986) suggests that the former explanation is unlikely, although a role for specific hemimethylated sites cannot be excluded. A related possibility is that the NCOR-binding proteins are stably bound and propagated (see Berg *et al.*, 1986) and are themselves modified during the passage of the replication fork, with the effect that the modified proteins inhibit new initiation events at the associated origin.

Another possibility is that the recognition event may take advantage of the structural properties of sister-chromatid regions, since sister chromatids can be present only in replicated DNA. Suppose that, as in BPV, there are two NCOR sites associated with each origin. Only replicons that have "fired" will contain four NCOR sites, two on each sister chromatid. Perhaps, for example, the negative, *trans*-acting factor is a tetrameric protein that requires NCOR occupancy of all four subunits for effective inhibition of origin function (Fig. 3). Repressor action will therefore be limited to those chromosomal regions that having been replicated, now contain the four associated NCOR sites required for repressor binding. This proposal seems to clearly predict that newly replicated BPV daughters may be held together as paired minichromosomes. At some time after S phase, all tetramers would presumably have to be removed or inactivated (e.g., by a general modification or a proteolysis system) to reset the system for a new round of replication in the next cell cycle.

Our conclusion that specific *cis*-acting sequences mediate a negative control of replication seems to contrast with some of the observations of Harland and Laskey (1980), who were the first to approach this problem experimentally by demonstrating that most circular DNA molecules microinjected into *Xenopus* embryos will replicate just once per cell cycle, independent of particular DNA sequences. Ironically, not only con-

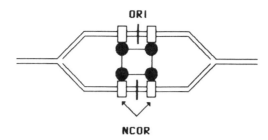

Figure 3. Schematic model for replication control. Shown is a possible arrangement of NCOR sequences and replication origins within a replicating region of the genome. Paired NCOR sequences are associated with each origin. Replication duplicates the NCOR sites, creating a tetrameric recognition site for factors that negatively control DNA replication (●). The assembly of this complex renders the associated origin unable to function in the initiation of DNA replication.

trol but also initiation of replication are independent of sequence in *Xenopus* embryos. Thus, in early embryogenesis in frog embryos, replication initiation can occur independently of sequence when initiation factors seem to be in excess; if negative modulators are also in excess, they too might function independently of sequence. This is not surprising, since most DNA-binding proteins have nonspecific affinities for DNA. What is surprising is that once bound to nonspecific sites, the replication-initiation and -control elements can apparently perform their functions efficiently and independently of DNA sequence.

4.3. Gene Amplification

Gene amplification probably occurs when a limited chromosomal region undergoes multiple rounds of DNA synthesis within a single cell cycle. It can therefore be viewed as a localized breakdown in the mechanisms that control DNA replication (Alt *et al.*, 1978; Botchan *et al.*, 1978; Roberts and Axel, 1982; Roberts *et al.*, 1983; Mariani and Schimke, 1984). In unusual circumstances, gene amplication occurs as a normal regulated developmental event associated with a rapid requirement for the product of the amplified gene(s) (Brown and Dawid, 1986; Spradling, 1981; Glover *et al.*, 1982). These cases may also be interpreted in terms of negative control to suggest that the cell possesses a mechanism to bypass the negative control of replication for the amplified genes.

Evidence is emerging that suggests that the cell also possesses a non-specific bypass mechanism that permits the reinitiation of replication under unusual circumstances on all DNA sequences (Varshavsky, 1981; Mariani and Schimke, 1984; Woodcock and Cooper, 1981). It has been known for some years that bacteria will reinitiate replication from the normal replication origin following treatments that impede the progress of the replication fork (e.g., thymidine starvation) (Pritchard and Lark, 1964). Eukaryotic cells will also reinitiate DNA replication over much of the genome following treatment with similar mutagenic agents, including hydroxyurea, ultraviolet light, and various other carcinogens (Lavi, 1981; Tlsty *et al.*, 1984; Mariani and Schimke, 1984). Associated with their abilities to impede DNA replication is the fact that all these agents are also mutagenic; hence, DNA replicated in the presence of these agents is likely to be a very unfaithful copy of the parental DNA. Perhaps the simplest way to repair the accumulated damage is to rereplicate the affected chromosomal regions when the mutagenic agent is removed and then to preserve only those nascent DNA molecules still attached to the main chromosome axis via base-pairing to the parental DNA strands. We interpret the decision to non-specifically reinitiate DNA replication as a kind of eukaryotic S.O.S. response to severe mutagenic damage; this may be mediated by a generalized removal of the negative controls on DNA replication.

4.4. Relation to the Inactive Mating-Type Cassettes in Yeast

While the molecular properties of the BPV NCOR system described herein may seem unusual, there are striking similarities to the control of the inactive mating-type cassettes of yeast (see reviews by Nasmyth, 1982; Klar *et al.*, 1985). Both systems control activity from a promoter (in yeast) or a replication origin (in BPV) located a considerable distance from two *cis*-acting negative control sites (E and I in yeast; NCOR I and II in BPV), which are themselves a considerable distance apart. Both types of *cis*-acting control sites are associated with activity of autonomously replicating sequences (or PMSs), and both are regulated by *trans*-acting elements (SIRs) for yeast; E1 for BPV. Most important, both systems regulate an activity that is permissible once and only once per cell generation. Replication must occur for SIR to inactivate the homothallic mating left (HML) or homothallic mating right (HMR) promoters (Miller and Nasmyth, 1984); similarly, we presume that replication must occur to inactivate replication origins. For replication control, repression must be relaxed once per cell cycle. While it is known that mating-type switching usually occurs once per cell cycle, direct evidence for a transient period of relaxed control at the inactive mating cassette (analogous to the activation of an origin) is lacking at present; however, this analogy predicts its existence. The observation that unregulated homothallic (HO) overexpression results in no apparent change in the pattern of mating-type switching (I. Herskowitz, personal communication) suggests that the inactive cassette is only rarely "competent" for switching. A similar relationship between the control of DNA replication and the control of the inactive cassettes has been pointed out and discussed extensively by Nasmyth (1982).

References

Alt, F. W., Kellems, R. E., Bertino, J. R., and Schimke, R. T., 1978, Selective multiplication of dihydrofolate reductase genes in methotrexate resistant variants of cultured murine cells, *J. Biol. Chem.* **252**:1357–1370.

Ariga, H., and Sugano, S., 1983, Initiation of simian virus 40 DNA replication *in vitro, J. Virol.* **48**:481–491.

Berg, L., Singh, K., and Botchan, M., 1986, Complementation of a BPV low copy number mutant: Evidence for a temporal requirement of the complementing gene, *Mol. Cell. Biol.* (in press).

Blumenthal, A. B., Kriegstein, H. J., and Hogness, D. S., 1973, The units of DNA replication in *Drosophila melanogaster* chromosomes, *Cold Spring Harbor Symp. Quant. Biol.* **38**:205–223.

Botchan, M., Topp, W., and Sambrook, J., 1978, Studies on simian virus 40 excision from cellular chromosomes, *Cold Spring Harbor Symp. Quant. Biol.* **43**:708–720.

Brown, D. D., and Dawid, I. B., 1986, Specific gene amplification in oocytes, *Science* **160**:272–280.

Chen, E.Y., Howley, P.M., Levinson, A. D., and Seeburg, P., 1982, The primary structure and genetic organization of the bovine papilloma-virus type I genome, *Nature (London)* **299**:529–534.

Colbere-Garapin, F., Horodniceanu, F., Kourilsky, P., and Garapin, A. C., 1981, A new dominant hybrid selective marker for higher eukaryotic cells, *J. Mol. Biol.* **150**:1–14.

DeLucia, A. L., Deb, S., Partin, K., and Tegtmeyer, P., 1986, Functional interactions of the simian virus 40 core origin of replication with flanking regulatory sequences, *J. Virol.* **57**:138–144.

DiMaio, D., Treisman, R., and Maniatis, T., 1982, Bovine papilloma virus vector that propagates as a plasmid in both mouse and bacterial cells, *Proc. Natl. Acad. Sci. U.S.A.* **79**:4030–4034.

DuBridge, R. B., Lusky, M., Botchan, M. R., and Calos, M. P., 1985, Amplification of a bovine papillomavirus–simian virus 40 chimera, *J. Virol.* **56**:625–627.

Glover, D. M., Zaha, A., Stocker, A. J., Santelli, R. V., Pueyo, M. T., deToledo, S. M., and Lara, F. J. S., 1982, Gene amplification in *Rhynchosciara* salivary gland chromosomes, *Proc. Natl. Acad. Sci. U.S.A.* **79**:2947–2951.

Gluzman, Y., 1981, SV40-transformed simian cells support the replication of early SV40 mutants, *Cell* **23**:175–182.

Hand, R., 1978, Eukaryotic DNA: Organization of the genome for replication, *Cell* **15**:317–325.

Harland, R. M., and Laskey, R. A., 1980, Regulation replication of DNA microinjected into eggs of *Xenopus laevis, Cell* **21**:761–771.

Heilman, C. A., Engel, L., Lowy, D. R., and Howley, P. M., 1982, Virus specific transcription in bovine papillomavirus transformed mouse cells, *Virology* **119**:22–34.

Jimenez, A., and Davies, Y., 1980, Expression of a transposable antibiotic resistance element in *Saccharomyces, Nature (London)* **287**:869–871.

Keshet, I., Lieman-Hurwitz, J., and Cedar, H., 1986, DNA methylation affects the formation of active chromatin, *Cell* **44**:535–543.

Klar, A. J. S., Strathern, J. N., and Hicks, J. B., 1985, Developmental pathways in yeast, in: *Microbial Development* (R. Losick and L. Shapiro, eds.), Cold Spring Harbor Laboratories, Cold Spring Harbor, New York, pp. 151–195.

Lavi, S., 1981, Carcinogen mediated amplification of viral DNA sequences in SV40 transformed Chinese hamster embryo cells, *Proc. Natl. Acad. Sci. U.S.A.* **78**:6144–6148.

Lancaster, W. D., 1981, Apparent lack of integration of bovine papilloma virus DNA in virus-induced equine and bovine tumor cells and virus transformed mouse cells, *Virology* **108**:251–255.

Law, M.-F., Lowy, D. R., Dvoretzky, J., and Howley, P. M., 1981, Mouse cells transformed by bovine papillomavirus contain only extra-chromosomal viral DNA sequences, *Proc. Natl. Acad. Sci. U.S.A.* **78**:2727–2731.

Li, J. J., and Kelly, T. J., 1984, Simian virus 40 DNA replication *in vitro, Proc. Natl. Acad. Sci. U.S.A.* **81**:6973–6977.

Lowy, D. R., Dvoretzky, I., Shober, R., Law, M.-F., Engel, L., and Howley, P. M., 1980, *In vitro* tumorigenic transformation by a defined sub-genomic fragment of bovine papilloma virus DNA, *Nature (London)* **287**:72–74.

Lusky, M., and Botchan, M., 1981, Inhibition of SV40 replication in simian cells by specific pBR322 DNA sequences, *Nature (London)* **293**:79–81.

Lusky, M., and Botchan, M., 1984, Characterization of the bovine papillomavirus plasmid maintenance sequences, *Cell* **36**:391–401.

Lusky, M., and Botchan, M., 1985, Genetic analysis of bovine papillomavirus type 1 *trans*-acting replication factors, *J. Virol.* **53**:955–965.

Lusky, M., and Botchan, M., 1986, Transient replication of BPV-1 plasmids: Cis and trans requirements, *Proc. Natl. Acad. Sci. U.S.A.* (in press).

Lusky, M., Berg, L., Weiher, H., and Botchan, M., 1983, Bovine papilloma virus contains an activator of gene expression at the distal end of the early transcription unit, *Mol. Cell. Biol.* **3**:1108–1122.

Meyers, R., and Tjian, R., 1980, Construction and analysis of simian virus 40 origins defective in tumor antigen binding and DNA replication, *Proc. Natl. Acad. Sci. U.S.A.* **77**:6491–6495.

Miller, A. M., and Nasmyth, K. A., 1984, Role of DNA replication in the repression of silent mating type loci in yeast, *Nature (London)* **312**:247–251.

Muriani, B., and Schimke, R., 1984, Gene amplification in a simple cell cycle in Chinese hamster ovary cells, *J. Biol. Chem.* **258**:1901–1910.

Nasmyth, K. A., 1982, Molecular genetics of yeast mating type, *Annu. Rev. Genet.* **16**:439–500.

Pritchard, R., and Lark, K., 1984, Induction of replication by thymine starvation at the chromosome origin in *E. coli*, *J. Mol. Biol.* **9**:288–307.

Rao, P. N., and Johnson, R. T., 1970, Mammalian cell fusion: Studies on the regulation of DNA synthesis and mitosis, *Nature (London)* **225**:159–164.

Roberts, J., and Axel, R., 1982, Gene amplification and gene correction in somatic cells, *Cell* **29**:109–119.

Roberts, J., and Weintraub, H., 1986, Negative control of DNA replication in composite SV40–bovine papilloma virus plasmids, *Cell* (in press).

Roberts, J., Buck, L., and Axel, R., 1983, A structure for amplified DNA, *Cell* **33**:53–63.

Roman, A., and Dulbecco, R., 1975, Fate of polyoma form I DNA during replication, *J. Virol.* **16**:70–74.

Sarver, N., Byrne, J. C., and Howley, P. M., 1982, Transformation and replication in mouse cells of a bovine papillomavirus–pML2 plasmid vector that can be rescued in bacteria, *Proc. Natl. Acad. Sci. U.S.A.* **79**:7147–7151.

Sarver, N., Rabson, M. S., Yang, Y.-C., Byrne, J. C., and Howley, P. M., 1984, Localization and analysis of bovine papillomavirus type 1 transforming functions, *J. Virol.* **52**:377–388.

Southern, P. J., and Berg, P., 1982, Transformation of mammalian cells to antibiotic resistance with a bacterial gene under control of the SV40 early region promoter, *J. Mol. Appl. Genet.* **1**:327–341.

Spalholz, B. A., Yang, Y. C., and Howley, P. M., 1985, Transactivation of a bovine papillomavirus transcriptional regulatory element by the E2 gene product, *Cell* **42**:183–191.

Spradling, A., 1981, The origin and amplification of two chromosomal domains containing *Drosophila* chorion genes, *Cell* **27**:193–201.

Stenlund, A., Zabielski, J., Ahola, H., Moreno-Lopez, J., and Petterson, U., 1985, The messenger RNAs from the transforming region of bovine papillomavirus type 1, *J. Mol. Biol.* **182**:541–554.

Tegtmeyer, P., 1972, Simian virus 40 deoxyribonucleic acid synthesis: The viral replicon, *J. Virol.* **10**:591–598.

Tjian, R., 1978, The binding site on SV40 DNA for a T antigen-related protein, *Cell* **13**:165–180.

Tlsty, T., Brown, P., and Schimke, R., 1984, UV radiation facilitates methotrexate resistance and amplification of the dihydrofolate reductase gene in cultured 3T6 mouse cells, *Mol. Cell. Biol.* **4**:1050–1056.

Tsui, L.-C., Breitman, M. L., Siminovitch, L., and Buchwald, M., 1982, Persistence of freely replicating SV40 recombinant molecules carrying a selectable marker in permissive simian cells, *Cell* **30**:499–508.

Varshavsky, A., 1981, On the possibility of metabolic control of replicon "mis-firing":

Relationship to emergence of malignant phenotypes in mammalian cell lineages, *Proc. Natl. Acad. Sci. U.S.A.* **78:**3673–3677.

Waldeck, W., Rosel, F., and Dengraf, H., 1984, Origin of replication in episomal bovine papilloma virus type I DNA isolated from transformed cell, *EMBO J.* **31:**2173–2178.

Woodcock, D., and Cooper, I., 1981, Evidence for double replication of chromosomal DNA segments as a general consequence of DNA replication inhibition, *Cancer Res.* **41:**2483–2490.

4

DNA Supercoiling as a Regulator of Bacterial Gene Expression

MARTIN GELLERT and ROLF MENZEL

1. Introduction

Studies of gene expression have advanced to a stage at which we can ask quite detailed questions about the factors that influence transcription and the ways in which these factors interact with each other. Such factors include not only the specific proteins that bind to regulatory sites on DNA, but also more subtle aspects of DNA structure, such as local bending, Z-DNA regions, and palindromic sequences.

The supercoiling of DNA has been of great interest to us and other people because of its possible role as a transcription regulator. An attractive feature of DNA supercoiling in this role is its transmission over long distances in a DNA chain. A topoisomerase could act on DNA at one location to alter its superhelicity, and the torsional change would be effective over many kilobases of DNA. In a circular plasmid, changes in supercoiling are likely to be sensed throughout the whole molecule. In a chromosomal structure, either in eukaryotes or in bacteria, DNA loops emerge from a central structure that constrains the base of the loops. Each loop, ranging from 50 to 100 kilobases in length, can therefore be independently supercoiled, with the constraining core playing the role that would be taken by the circular continuity of the DNA chain in a plasmid. From this point of view, it becomes immaterial that bacterial chromosomes are circular while eukaryotic chromosomes are generally linear; the possibility

MARTIN GELLERT and ROLF MENZEL • Laboratory of Molecular Biology, National Institute of Diabetes, and Digestive and Kidney Diseases, National Institutes of Health, Bethesda, Maryland 20892. *Present address for* R. M.: Department of Research and Development, DuPont de Nemours, Wilmington, Delaware 19898.

of independently altered supercoiling of individual loops, and the trans-missibility of torsional stress throughout a loop, exists in either case. We may note the tantalizing observation that in eukaryotic chromosomes, topoisomerase II has been found to be highly concentrated in the chro-mosome scaffold structure (Earnshaw and Heck, 1985), so that topolo-gical alterations may be produced at the base of the loops preferentially. Although possible effects of supercoiling on eukaryotic gene expression have been widely discussed, a treatment of this complex subject would take us too far afield. The remainder of this chapter will therefore be devoted to prokaryotic systems.

How might we expect DNA supercoiling to affect transcription? DNA is found to be negatively supercoiled in all organisms investigated so far [with the exception of one species of thermophilic archaebacterium (see Nadal *et al.*, 1986)]; the twisting stress in such a DNA molecule can be partly relieved by local unwinding of the double helix. A possible rela-tionship between transcription initiation and DNA unwinding was uncov-ered some years ago, when it was found that the binding of *Escherichia coli* RNA polymerase leads to the unwinding of DNA by about one heli-cal turn (Saucier and Wang, 1972). These measurements were subse-quently refined and extended to show that an unwound loop of about the same size travels with the advancing polymerase throughout RNA chain elongation (Gamper and Hearst, 1982). The results fit naturally into the standard kinetic model of RNA polymerase action (recently reviewed by McClure, 1985), in which the initial reversible attachment of the enzyme to a promoter site is followed by the irreversible, and frequently slower, formation of an "open" complex in which the DNA is locally unwound. The open complex is a necessary intermediate in transcription.

This kinetic sequence assigns an obvious role to DNA supercoiling. Increased negative supercoiling would facilitate open-complex formation by reducing the energetic cost of DNA unwinding and would thus tend to speed up transcription initiation. In fact, the first studies in this area found an enhancement of transcription by supercoiling: Transcription from ϕX174 replicative-form DNA and from both of the early promoters of phage λ is increased when the DNA is supercoiled (Hayashi and Hayashi, 1971; Botchan *et al.*, 1973).

Later work has shown that the effects of supercoiling are much more varied and complex than the first studies revealed (see the recent review by Drlica, 1984). Most of the reported results come from *in vivo* exper-iments and generally require inferences from indirect methods used to change the level of intracellular supercoiling. Most of this work has been done in *E. coli* and *Salmonella typhimurium*. Here, the balance of supercoiling appears to be set, to a first approximation, by the competing activities of DNA gyrase, which increases the superhelicity, and topoisomerase I, which returns the DNA to a more relaxed state. Changes in supercoiling are produced by interfering with the activity, or altering the amount, of one enzyme or the other. Gyrase activity can be reduced by specific inhibitors of either the A or the B subunit or by temperature-sensitive mutations that have been isolated in both the *gyrA* and the *gyrB* genes. Although the quinolone antibiotics that inhibit the DNA break–join activity of the A subunit (compounds such as nalidixic acid, oxolinic acid, and norfloxacin) have been widely used, they give results that are not always easy to interpret, because they kill cells at concentrations 10- to 100-fold lower than those needed to inhibit intracellular DNA supercoiling. The lethal effect is still mediated by DNA gyrase, but may involve the well-known quinolone-induced breakage of DNA by DNA gyrase rather than any alteration of superhelicity. The coumarin antibiotics (e.g., coumermycin A_1, novobiocin), which act on the gyrase B subunit, seem to affect the supercoiling activity alone in a simpler manner.

Studies with these inhibitors have shown that expression of different genes is affected very differently (Drlica, 1984). Some genes are strongly repressed when DNA gyrase is inhibited (10- to 20-fold alterations are not rare), some are activated, and most are relatively unaffected. Earlier studies that focused on individual genes could not yield reliable estimates of how many genes fell into each class. We recently tested operon fusions of shotgun-cloned *E. coli* promoters to the galactokinase structural gene and found that roughly 15–20% are greatly inhibited by blocking gyrase activity, a similar number are activated, and the rest are more or less unaffected (Menzel and Gellert, 1987).

No specific inhibitors are known for bacterial topoisomerase I, nor have convenient temperature-sensitive mutants been available. Transcription studies in *E. coli* and *Salmonella* have used either partly defective mutants or deletions of the *topA* gene. Unlike DNA gyrase, topoisomerase I is not absolutely essential for viability, so even deletion mutants can survive. Results in *E. coli* are complicated by the fact that mutants totally lacking topoisomerase I grow very slowly and are soon overgrown by cells containing secondary mutations that restore supercoiling to a lower level. Some of these "compensating mutations" map in *gyrA* or *gyrB* and lead to reduced gyrase activity (DiNardo *et al.*, 1982; Pruss *et al.*, 1982;

Gellert *et al.*, 1982); others map in a third locus named *toc*, for which no function is yet known (Raji *et al.*, 1985).

Transcription studies with *topA* mutants have therefore been done mainly in *Salmonella* or in *E. coli* strains only partly defective in topoisomerase I. These studies actually began with the work of Margolin and his colleagues (Mukai and Margolin, 1963) on the so-called *supX* mutants of *S. typhimurium*, which were originally identified as suppressing a promoter-defective mutation (*leu*-500) in the leucine operon and were later shown to also change the expression of several other genes. The *supX* mutations are now known to lie in the *topA* gene and to result in a lowered or absent topoisomerase I activity. This defect increases the average level of supercoiling in the cells; the *leu*-500 promoter, which is poorly expressed at normal levels of supercoiling, is now restored to higher activity, and of course other promoters are likewise affected. These studies are complementary to those in which gyrase activity is inhibited; both types of experiments show that changes in supercoiling have a multiplicity of effects on transcription.

2. Results and Discussion

Our own work in this field began with the supposition that if DNA superhelicity has pleiotropic effects on gene expression, cells are likely to have special regulatory mechanisms for controlling the level of supercoiling. We therefore decided to look at the expression of the *gyrA* and *gyrB* genes themselves. We pulse-labeled *E. coli* cells with radioactive methionine and then isolated the gyrase A and gyrase B proteins with the help of specific antibodies. We were then able to measure the rate of synthesis of both proteins under a variety of conditions. It was easy to show that treatment of cells with coumermycin A_1 or novobiocin, at concentrations high enough to block intracellular gyrase activity, resulted in a large increase in the production of gyrase; the rates of synthesis of both subunits were increased about 10-fold (Menzel and Gellert, 1983). Similarly, in cells containing a temperature-sensitive mutation in the *gyrB* gene, synthesis of gyrase A and gyrase B proteins was greatly increased at 42°C. All these treatments were expected to decrease the level of DNA supercoiling; the most plausible explanation for the increased gyrase synthesis was that it was a response to this change in superhelicity.

Experiments in an *in vitro* system allowed us to show that this interpretation was correct. The advantage of cell-free experiments is that the topological state of the input DNA can be controlled independently of other changes in the system. In a protein-synthesizing extract programmed by plasmids containing the *gyrA* and *gyrB* genes and promoters, synthesis of the gyrase subunits was much greater when the plasmids were presented in relaxed form than when they were supercoiled. A further increase was seen if novobiocin was added to prevent the gyrase activity present in the extract from acting on the relaxed DNA. The overall increase, from supercoiled DNA to relaxed DNA in the presence of novobiocin, was about 100-fold (Menzel and Gellert, 1983).

These results immediately suggested that DNA supercoiling in *E. coli* is homeostatically controlled. When supercoiling drops to a low level, gyrase synthesis is increased, leading to a higher supercoiling activity in the cells. When the level of supercoiling is too high, gyrase synthesis decreases. How does the regulation of the competing enzyme, topoisomerase I, fit into this control mechanism? This system was investigated by Tse-Dinh (1985), who was able to show that expression of the *topA* gene is also regulated by DNA superhelicity, but in exactly the opposite way from the regulation of DNA gyrase. Synthesis of topoisomerase I is greatest when the DNA is highly supercoiled, which again tends to restore superhelicity to a more intermediate level. Thus, the amounts of the two enzymes are adjusted to maintain an intermediate level of supercoiling. This is at least a partial answer to the question of how supercoiling is regulated, although it does not take into account possible modulations of the *activity* of both enzymes in the cell or the existence of at least one other minor DNA-relaxing activity (topoisomerase III).

These results bring into sharper focus a second general question, raised earlier in this chapter: Why is the expression of different genes affected differently by changes in supercoiling? More specifically, why are some genes induced by DNA relaxation?

Once more, the gyrase genes have served as a convenient system for studying this issue. We have shown (R. Menzel and M. Gellert, manuscript in preparation) that relaxation induction does not require an extensive region of DNA. Deletions or transposon insertions upstream of *gyrB* do not alter this form of control unless they come very near [within 100 base pairs (bp)] the structural gene. Guided by this observation, we inserted short regions containing the 5' ends of the *gyrA* or the *gyrB* gene and their immediate leader sequences into plasmids that carry the *galK* structural gene, arranged so that the inserts form operon fusions. Here again, sequences extending about 100 bp upstream of *gyrA* or *gyrB* were long enough to give relaxation-induced expression of galactokinase in cells carrying the plasmids. These sequences therefore contain the respective promoters and all the sequence information necessary for this type of regulation. The promoter sites are in fact readily identifiable by examination of the sequence.

We were then in a position to find out exactly how much of each of the two sequences was required. We constructed deletions that reached into the promoter regions from the upstream or downstream sides and further tested plasmids that still expressed galactokinase *in vivo* for their response to inhibition of gyrase activity. The results of the deletion analysis can be summarized as follows:

1. Deletions from the upstream side can reach well into the *gyrA* or *gyrB* promoter without upsetting relaxation induction. Even deletions as close as 3 bp to the −10 consensus region still behave like the parent promoter. The overall strength of the promoter is modulated by the sequences that have been adventitiously brought into the −35 region and varies in an understandable way according to their fit to the −35 consensus, but relaxation induction is independent of changes in that region.
2. Deletions from the downstream side begin to affect expression when they approach to within 3–5 bases downstream of the transcription start. Many of these deletions lower the basal level of galactokinase synthesis and in parallel *increase* the factor of induction by gyrase inhibition.
3. A double deletion of the *gyrA* promoter that retains only 21 bp, including the −10 consensus and the transcription start, is still normally induced by DNA relaxation.

In considering the implications of these results, one must also take into account that apart from the very good fit to the −10 consensus sequence in both cases (TATAAT for *gyrA*, TAAAAT for *gyrB*), there is no visible homology between the two promoter sequences in this region. Thus, there is no unique sequence responsible for relaxation induction, unless it is the −10 consensus itself, and this seems unlikely because the same sequence occurs in promoters that are not relaxation induced.

What other possible explanations are there for this phenomenon? One proposed model (Borowiec and Gralla, 1985) depends on the natural variation in spacing between the -10 and -35 consensus regions. This spacing varies from 15 to 20 nucleotides in *E. coli* promoters, with the preferred value being 17 or 18. Because RNA polymerase has to contact both regions, there could also be a preferred value of the angle around the DNA helix between the -10 and -35 regions. Extra-long spacers would then make this angle too large, but it could be restored by greater negative supercoiling of the DNA; in extra-short spacers, the angle would be too small and could be improved by decreased supercoiling. Although this model has attractive features, it is not compatible with our deletion results. The upstream deletions can remove the original -35 sequence and replace it with others that fit the consensus more or less well and have a variety of spacings from the -10 region, all without significantly changing relaxation induction. Another possibility is that other proteins besides RNA polymerase are involved in this form of regulation. It should be emphasized that this alternative cannot yet be ruled out because we have not yet succeeded in obtaining relaxation induction of either gyrase promoter with purified RNA polymerase alone, but only in whole cells or in crude extracts.

An alternative that we find more appealing, however, is that relaxation induction can be explained by invoking an aspect of transcription initiation that we have not yet discussed. RNA polymerase does not only make long RNA molecules; it also generates some so-called "abortive" transcripts 2–10 nucleotides long. The proportion of abortive transcripts to full-length ones depends on the promoter sequence. For a few promoters that have been identified, the large majority of transcription starts result in abortive transcripts (Stefano and Gralla, 1979; Munson and Reznikoff, 1981). Abortive transcription does not prevent renewed initiation by the same RNA polymerase molecule, because the σ subunit is not normally released until RNA chain elongation has gone somewhat further. An RNA polymerase molecule can thus make several attempts at initiating a full-length transcript; the overall rate of messenger RNA synthesis will be diminished by the fraction of failed attempts.

How could this process affect relaxation induction? Before RNA polymerase can reinitiate, the abortive transcript must be released. This step would be highly sensitive to DNA supercoiling, because the RNA fragment would presumably be held in an RNA–DNA hybrid structure as a miniature "R-loop." Such R-loops are expected to be greatly stabilized by DNA supercoiling. *Release* of the RNA fragment would be faster in relaxed DNA, and the rate of reinitiation could be correspondingly faster. Some circumstantial evidence in favor of this model comes from studies of the *lac*-UV5 mutant promoter, which is known to make an abnormally high proportion of abortive transcripts and which is also, at least under some conditions, stimulated by DNA relaxation (Sanzey, 1979). Another line of evidence comes from the deletion experiments cited above. Those downstream deletions, ending within the first few bases of the transcribed region, that most strongly reduce the basal level of *in vivo* transcription are also the most strongly induced by DNA relaxation. We suggest that these sequence changes may affect the synthesis and release of abortive transcripts and, in parallel, the extent of stimulation by DNA relaxation. Experiments to challenge this interpretation are now in progress.

Finally, we want to point out that these modulations of steady-state transcriptional activity are by no means the only regulatory effects of changes in supercoiling. When *E. coli* cells are treated with coumermycin, there is transient induction of a group of proteins that turns out to be essentially the same group induced by heat shock (Travers and Mace, 1982). The two phenomena are closely related, because *htpR* mutants that do not respond to heat shock also fail to show a shock response to coumermycin (Yura *et al.*, 1984). Nevertheless, gyrase induction is normal in these mutants, thus emphasizing that the two effects of supercoiling alterations are distinct (unpublished observations). Coumermycin treatment also leads to slow activation of the S.O.S. response; here again, it can be shown that gyrase induction is still normal in *recA* mutants that are deficient in the S.O.S. response (unpublished results). There are evidently several different ways in which the topological state of DNA can influence gene expression and genetic control circuits in bacterial cells.

References

Borowiec, J. A., and Gralla, J. D., 1985, Supercoiling response of the *lac* p^s promoter *in vitro*, *J. Mol. Biol.* **184**:587–598.

Botchan, P., Wang, J. C., and Echols, H., 1973, Effect of circularity and superhelicity on transcription from bacteriophage λ DNA, *Proc. Natl. Acad. Sci. U.S.A.* **70**:3077–3081.

DiNardo, S., Voelkel, K. A., Sternglanz, R., Reynolds, A. E., and Wright, A., 1982, *Escherichia coli* DNA topoisomerase I mutants have compensatory mutations in DNA gyrase genes, *Cell* **31**:43–51.

Drlica, K., 1984, Biology of bacterial deoxyribonucleic acid topoisomerases, *Microbiol. Rev.* **1984**:273-289.

Earnshaw, W. C., and Heck, M. M. S., 1985, Localization of topoisomerase II in mitotic chromosomes, *J. Cell Biol.* **100**:1716-1725.

Gamper, H. B., and Hearst, J. E., 1982, A topological model for transcription based on unwinding angle analysis of *E. Coli* RNA polymerase binary, initiation and ternary complexes, *Cell* **29**:81-90.

Gellert, M., Menzel, R., Mizuuchi, K., O'Dea, M. H., and Friedman, D. I., 1982, Regulation of DNA supercoiling in *Escherichia coli*, *Cold Spring Harbor Symp. Quant. Biol.* **47**:763-767.

Hayashi, Y., and Hayashi, M., 1971, Template activities of the ϕX174 replicative allomorphic deoxyribonucleic acids, *Biochemistry* **10**:4212-4218.

McClure, W. R., 1985, Mechanism and control of transcription initiation in prokaryotes, *Annu. Rev. Biochem.* **54**:171-204.

Menzel, R., and Gellert, M., 1983, Regulation of the genes for *E. Coli* DNA gyrase: Homeostatic control of DNA supercoiling, *Cell* **34**:105-113.

Menzel, R., and Gellert, M., 1987, Fusions of the *E. coli gyrA* and *gyrB* control regions to the galactokinase gene are inducible by DNA relaxation, *J. Bacteriol.* (submitted)

Mukai, F. H., and Margolin, P., 1963, Analysis of unlinked suppressors of an 0° mutation in *Salmonella, Proc. Natl. Acad. Sci. U.S.A.* **50**:140-148.

Munson, L. M., and Reznikoff, W. S., 1981, Abortive initiation and long ribonucleic acid synthesis, *Biochemistry* **20**:2081-2085.

Nadal, M., Mirambeau, G., Forterre, P., Reiter, W., and Duguet, M., 1986, Positively supercoiled DNA exists *in vivo, Nature (London)* **321**:256-258.

Pruss, G. J., Manes, S. H., and Drlica, K., 1982, *Escherichia coli* topoisomerase I mutants: Increased supercoiling is corrected by mutations near gyrase genes, *Cell* **31**:35-42.

Raji, A., Zabel, D. J., Laufer, C. S., and Depew, R. E., 1985, Genetic analysis of mutations that compensate for loss of *Escherichia coli* DNA topoisomerase I, *J. Bacteriol.* **162**:1173-1179.

Sanzey, B., 1979, Modulation of gene expression by drugs affecting deoxyribonucleic acid gyrase, *J. Bacteriol.* **138**:40-47.

Saucier, J. M., and Wang, J. C., 1972, Angular alteration of the DNA helix by *E. coli* RNA polymerase, *Nature New Biol.* **239**:167-170.

Stefano, J. E., and Gralla, J., 1979, Lac UV5 transcription *in vitro*: Rate limitation subsequent to formation of an RNA polymerase-DNA complex, *Biochemistry* **18**:1063-1067.

Travers, A. A., and Mace, H. A. F., 1982, The heat shock phenomenon in bacteria— A protection against DNA relaxation. *Heat Shock from Bacteria to Man* (M. J. Schlesinger, M. Ashburner, and A. Tissieres, eds.), Cold Spring Harbor Laboratory, Cold Spring Harbor, New York, pp. 127-130.

Tse-Dinh, Y. C., 1985, Regulation of the *Escherichia coli* DNA topoisomerase I gene by DNA supercoiling, *Nucleic Acid Res.* **13**:4751-4763.

Yura, T., Tobe, T., Ito, K., and Osawa, T., 1984, Heat shock regulatory gene (*htpR*) of *Escherichia coli* is required for growth at high temperature but is dispensable at low temperature, *Proc. Natl. Acad. Sci. U.S.A.* **81**:6803-6807.

5

Retrotransposition in Yeast

GERALD R. FINK

1. Introduction

The Ty elements of yeast are repetitive chromosomal elements capable of transposition, a nonhomologous recombination event that leads to insertion of an element at a new chromosomal site. The structure of Ty elements is similar to that of the endogenous proviruses found in vertebrates (Clare and Farabaugh, 1985; Mount and Rubin, 1985). Each element contains a large central portion of approximately 5.2 kilobases flanked by direct repeats of about 330 base pairs (bp) called δ or long terminal repeat (LTR) sequences (Fig. 1). Ty elements are repeated about 30–40 times per haploid genome and are found in variable chromosomal locations in different strains.

2. Experiments

We analyzed Ty transposition by studying the behavior of one element, TyH3, and replacing its promoter with the *GAL1* promoter (Boeke *et al.*, 1985). In intact Ty elements, a promoter in the 5′ LTR is responsible for the initiation of a transcript that begins in the 5′ LTR and terminates in the 3′ LTR. When TyH3 is fused to the *GAL1* promoter (plasmids containing this hybrid Ty are called pGTyH3), a Ty transcript with a normal 5′ end is produced. Substitution of the *GAL1* promoter for the

GERALD R. FINK • Whitehead Institute for Biomedical Research, Massachusetts Institute of Technology, Cambridge, Massachusetts 02142.

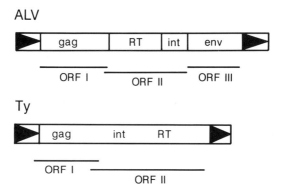

Figure 1. Comparison of avian leukosis virus (ALV) with Ty element. (RT) Reverse tran-scriptase; (int) integrase; (env) envelope; (ORF) open reading frame. The overall features of ALV are inferred from Rous sarcoma virus and those of Ty from the sequence of Clare and Farabaugh (1985).

Ty promoter in pGTyH3 stimulates transposition: Cells containing pGTyH3 show at least 100-fold enhancement of transposition when grown on galactose (induced for transposition) as compared with the frequency when grown on glucose (repressed for transposition).

The transposition frequency was monitored by reversion of an *his3* promoter deletion (Fig. 2). In this method, the cell contains two plasmids. The *donor* for transposition is the pGTyH3 plasmid, and the *recipient* is a plasmid that carries a *his3* gene the promoter of which is deleted. The cells containing these plasmids cannot grow in the absence of histidine because they have a deletion of the *his3* gene on the chromosome. If a Ty element inserts into the recipient plasmid, the defective *his3* gene on the plasmid becomes activated and the cell can grow on medium lacking histidine. Apparently, the Ty element has an enhancerlike sequence cap-able of activating transcription in the promoterless *his3* gene.

We marked the Ty element in pTyH3 with various DNA sequences and followed the transposition of this marked element from the donor to the recipient plasmid. We then isolated from yeast the recipient plasmid that confers the His[+] phenotype and analyzed it to determine the struc-ture of the Ty element that had transposed. The fate of a donor element that had been marked with an intron revealed the mechanism by which Ty elements transpose. Ty elements have no introns, so we inserted an intron plus its flanking exons derived from the gene for a yeast ribosomal

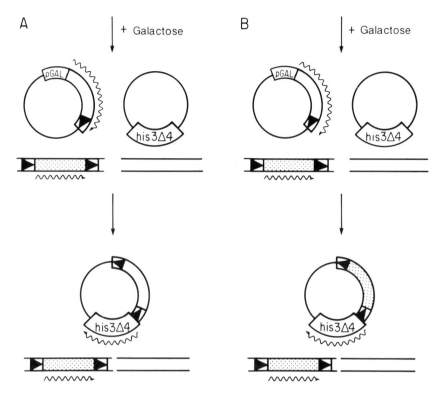

Figure 2. Catalysis of transposition in *trans* by TyH3. (▶) LTRs of the Ty. (A) The circular plasmid at top left is the donor pGTyH3. pGAL is the *GAL1* promoter attached to the Ty element, TyH3. The recipient plasmid to the right of TyH3 contains the *his3* promoter deletion. The stippled Ty represents one of the chromosomal Ty's. The diagram shows that induction of TyH3 transcription by galactose leads to transposition of TyH3. (B) Induction of transcription in pGTyH3 also leads to enhanced transposition of chromosomal Ty elements.

protein into TyH3. The transposition of this marked donor Ty element to the recipient plasmid resulted in removal of the intron. The intron was removed precisely by the rules of RNA splicing. This result means that Ty elements transpose DNA → RNA → DNA.

Yeast cells that contain the galactose-promoted Ty element and are induced for transposition have both reverse transcriptase activity and virus-like particles (Garfinkel *et al.*, 1985). The reverse transcriptase co-sediments with genomic length Ty RNA and a Ty-specified protein antigen in a particulate fraction. This complex is able to synthesize a full-length

Ty complementary DNA (cDNA), suggesting that reverse transcription of Ty RNA takes place in the particle. The particles can be observed in thin sections of Ty-transposition-induced cells and resemble the intracisternal A-type particles of the mouse and copia particles of *Drosophila*. The presence of reverse transcriptase and viruslike particles supports the idea that Ty elements and retroviruses share a common origin.

Not all the elements that transpose into the recipient *his3* plasmid are identical to the donor TyH3 (Boeke *et al.*, 1985). In fact, at least three distinct types of Ty elements (discussed below) are recovered after transposition is induced by growth on galactose. The differences can be revealed by hybridizing these newly transposed Ty's to a probe for the marker in the donor pGTyH3 in conjunction with restriction-enzyme analysis.

The first type of Ty element recovered is similar to the donor Ty, TyH3, except for the expected changes from reverse transcription. The second type fails to hybridize with the probe for the marker, and its restriction enzymes differ in many ways from those of the donor TyH3. These novel elements are likely to be reverse transcripts of chromosomal Ty's the retrotransposition of which was catalyzed *in trans* by the induction of the donor pGTyH3. This conclusion is supported by the fact that the frequency with which these novel elements appear is elevated approximately 100-fold by induction of TyH3. Furthermore, when the pattern of chromosomal Ty's is examined by Southern analysis before and after galactose induction of pGTyH3, glucose-grown cells show the same pattern as the uninduced starting strain, whereas galactose-grown cells show a dramatically altered distribution of Ty elements. Virtually every galactose-induced cell has a different distribution and an altered number of elements. Subsequent studies show that at least some of these new sites of Ty hybridization represent induced transposition of chromosomal elements to new chromosomal locations (Fig. 2).

The third type of recovered Ty element retains the hybridization marker placed in the donor element, but differs from the donor element in one or more restriction sites. These elements appear to be altered forms of the donor element. The alterations could arise either from mutations resulting from reverse transcription or from recombination between the cDNA of the donor elements and a cDNA encoded by one of the endogenous chromosomal elements (see Fig. 3).

The existence of an *spt3* mutation (Winston *et al.*, 1984a, b) that abolishes LTR–LTR transcription allows discrimination between the two models described above. Previous studies have shown that strains that con-

A. REPLICATION   B. RECOMBINATION WITH
    ERROR   ENDOGENOUS Ty's

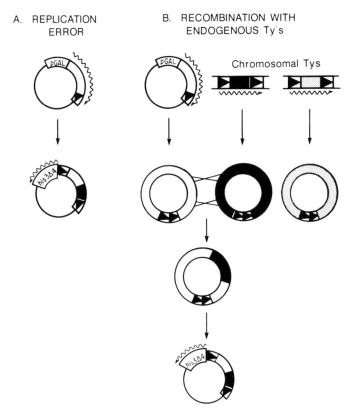

Figure 3. Two models to explain the generation of altered Ty's during transposition. (A) New sequences are generated by the mutagenic effects of reverse transcriptase. The plasmid contains the donor pGYyH3 as in Fig. 2. The plasmid below is an His⁺ derivative resulting from transposition of TyH3. The black segment represents new sequences found after transposition. (B) New sequences are generated by recombination between the donor Ty (white pGTyH3) and the chromosomal Ty (black) to produce a hybrid Ty element. The recombination event could take place during or after reverse transcription. The intermediates shown here are hypothetical and are based on the structures found for retroviruses.

tain the *spt3* mutation have no detectable full-length Ty transcript. This must mean that SPT3 is required for initiation of transcription at the 5' LTR of each of the chromosomal Ty's. The fact that pGTyH3 (which has the galactose promoter in place of the 5' LTR promoter) is the only Ty that produces a Ty transcript in *spt⁻* cells induced with galactose is consistent with this interpretation.

One can test whether recombination is responsible for the altered donor Ty's by comparing the structure of marked Ty elements that transpose in *SPT*⁺ and *spt3*⁻ strains. In *spt3*⁻ strains, there should be no copies of the chromosomal Ty cDNAs available for recombination with the donor TyH3 cDNA. We constructed isogenic *SPT*⁺ and *spt*⁻ strains, using the transformation integration and excision procedure, and induced for transposition. In the *SPT3* strains, about 30% of the transposed elements were altered donor types, whereas in *spt3*⁻ strains, fewer than 1% were of this type. This result means that the altered forms of the donor element were a result of recombination. The recombination events could occur during reverse transcription (if the partially completed cDNA hopped from the marked donor Ty template to an RNA derived from one of the chromosomal Tys) or after reverse transcription at the level of the cDNAs. Recombination events of this type have been described for retroviruses (Junghans *et al.*, 1982).

3. Speculation

These interactions between the donor Ty and the endogenous chromosomal elements during retrotransposition raise the possibility that Ty reverse transcriptase may, under some circumstances, reverse-transcribe normal cellular messages. The cDNAs resulting from reverse transcription could then recombine with the genomic copy of the gene. If the resident genomic copy contains an intron, then two crossovers, one on either side of the intron, would lead to loss of that intron. A diagrammatic representation of a sequence of events that could lead to the removal of an intron is shown in Fig. 4.

The presence of pseudogenes in mammalian cells has been explained as resulting from reverse transcription of cellular RNAs (Nishioka *et al.*, 1980). Pseudogenes are thought to represent integrated copies of reverse transcripts because they often lack a promoter and any introns present in the active copy and contain polyadenylic acid [poly(A)] stretches in the 3′ untranslated region that are absent from the active copy. Pseudogenes are often inactive because of mutations and are usually present in a different chromosomal location from the active copy. Surprisingly, *Saccharomyces cerevisiae* has few if any pseudogenes.

The presence of pseudogenes in mammalian cells and their apparent absence from *Saccharomyces* could be a consequence of the nature of the

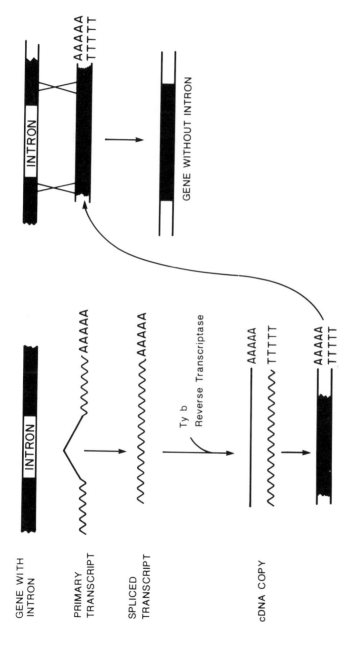

Figure 4. Loss of an intron by reverse transcription of a cellular messenger RNA. In this model, the reverse transcriptase encoded by the Ty b open reading frame catalyzes the formation of a cDNA from cellular message. This message is converted into a double-stranded form that recombines with the resident copy. The recombination event shown would lead to loss of the intron.

recombination process that leads to the integration of the cDNA. In mammalian cells, exogenous DNA introduced by transformation usually integrates by nonhomologous recombination, whereas in *Saccharomyces* it always integrates by homologous recombination. Nonhomologous recombination events in mammalian cells would integrate all the information in the message, including the poly(A), at new chromosomal sites. A cDNA integrated by nonhomologous recombination would have all the features of a pseudogene. In yeast, homologous recombination events would replace part of the resident active copy with homologous segments of the cDNA. Poly(A) stretches from the cDNA could not be integrated because they lack homology with the chromosomal copy. Homologous recombination between the resident copy and the cDNA would not lead to formation of a pseudogene at a site distinct from the active copy. In fact, the only evidence for recombination between the cDNA and the genomic copy would be the loss of an intron.

Many of the steps shown in Fig. 4 are not unreasonable in view of what is known about the fate of DNA molecules during transformation in *Saccharomyces*. Reverse transcription of a message would result in a single-stranded DNA (ssDNA) molecule. Previous work (Singh *et al.*, 1982) has shown that yeast can be efficiently transformed with ssDNA molecules containing a yeast autonomously replicating segment. Since subsequent isolation of the transforming DNA from yeast yields solely double-stranded molecules, it has been inferred that yeast has the ability to synthesize the second strand from single-stranded templates. In fact, recent experiments in my own laboratory have indicated that ssDNA is as efficient as double-stranded DNA (dsDNA) in integrative transformation. The presence of a system in yeast that converts ssDNA to dsDNA and a highly efficient homologous recombination pathway are compatible with the final steps shown in Fig. 4.

The most difficult steps to rationalize are the events that initiate reverse transcription of the cellular RNAs. Initiation by reverse transcriptase requires a primer. In retroviruses, the primer is a host transfer RNA (tRNA) that has homology with a sequence near the 5′ end of the retroviral RNA (Varmus, 1983). DNA synthesis begins by addition to the 3′ end of the tRNA. Although there is no obvious candidate for the primer of cellular RNA reverse transcription, it is possible that there are regions of cellular messages that have some homology with tRNAs and that this homology is sufficient to permit the priming reaction to proceed. Reverse transcriptase does not require extensive homology between the template and the tRNA primer. Only 16 bp at the 3′ terminus of tRNA^{trp} are bound to Rous sarcoma virus (Eiden *et al.*, 1976; Cordell *et al.*, 1979).

Another possible difficulty is the inaccessability of the cellular RNAs to the reverse transcriptase. In retroviruses, reverse transcription takes place in infecting particles, effectively isolating the reaction from other cellular components. The model in Fig. 4 could work if cellular messages are occasionally packaged, instead of Ty RNA. Alternatively, there could

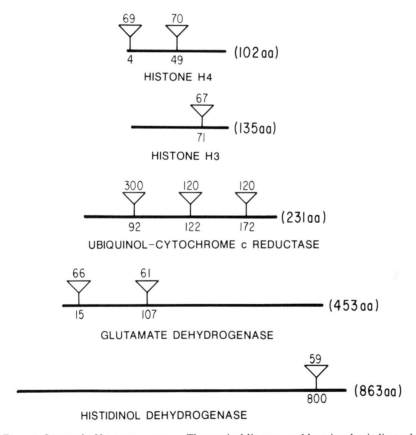

Figure 5. Introns in *Neurospora* genes. The vertical lines topped by triangles indicate the positions of the introns. The number above the triangle gives the size of the intron; the number below the intron gives the position relative to the 5′ A of the ATG. The number in parentheses is the number of amino acid residues in the protein. Sources for the data are as follows: histones—Woudt *et al.* (1983); ubiquinol-cytochrome *c* reductase—Harnisch *et al.* (1985); glutamate dehydrogenase—Kinnaird and Fincham (1983); histidinol dehydrogenase—Legerton and Yanofsky (1985).

be conditions under which reverse transcriptase is unassociated with particles. These conditions could occur when reverse transcriptase is overproduced or in mutants when packaging of the Ty RNA is defective.

Genes in *Saccharomyces* are generally devoid of introns; only the genes for some of the ribosomal proteins and actin have them. By contrast, many genes in *Neurospora* and Schizosaccharomyces contain introns. Figure 5 shows the location of introns of several *Neurospora* genes. It is interesting to note that the equivalent genes in *Saccharomyces* lack introns. The paucity of introns in *Saccharomyces* could be a result of the action of the Ty reverse transcriptase by the process shown in Fig. 4. Since most *Saccharomyces* genes are present in single copy, intron removal by Ty reverse transcriptase in haploid cells could never be corrected by gene conversion with an intron-containing copy. If this explanation for the difference between the structure of genes in *Saccharomyces* and *Neurospora* is correct, then one would expect neither retroviral elements nor reverse transcriptase in *Neurospora*.

References

Boeke, J. D., Garfinkel, D. J., Styles, C. A., and Fink, G. R., 1985, Ty elements transpose through an RNA intermediate, *Cell* **40**:491–500.

Clare, J., and Farabaugh, P., 1985, Nucleotide sequence of a yeast Ty element: Evidence for an unusual mechanism of gene expression, *Proc. Natl. Acad. Sci. U.S.A.* **82**:2829–2833.

Cordell, B., Swanstrom, R., Goodman, H. M., and Bishop, J. M., 1979, tRNA[trp] as primer for RNA-directed DNA polymerase: Structural determinants of function, *J. Biol. Chem.* **254**:1866–1874.

Eiden, J. J., Quade, K., and Nichols, J. L., 1976, Interaction of tryptophan transfer RNA with Rous sarcoma virus 355 RNA, *Nature (London)* **259**:245–247.

Garfinkel, D. J., Boeke, J. D., and Fink, G. R., 1985, Ty element transposition: Reverse transcriptase and virus-like particles, *Cell* **42**:507–517.

Harnisch, U., Weiss, H., and Sebald, W., 1985, The primary structure of the iron–sulfur subunit of ubiquinol-cytochrome c reductase from *Neurospora*, determined by cDNA and gene sequencing, *Eur. J. Biochem.* **149**:95–99.

Junghans, R. P., Boone, L. R., and Skalka, A. M., 1982, Retroviral DNA H structures: Displacement–assimilation model of recombination, *Cell* **30**:53–62.

Kinnaird, J. H., and Fincham, J. R. S., 1983, The complete nucleotide sequence of the *Neurospora crassa* am (NADP-specific glutamate dehydrogenase) gene, *Gene* **26**:253–260.

Legerton, T. L. and Yanofsky, C., 1985, Cloning and characterization of the multifunctional his-3 gene of *Neurospora crassa*, *Gene* **39**:129–140.

Mount, S. M., and Rubin, G. M., 1985, Complete nucleotide sequence of the *Drosophila* transposable element copia: Homology between copia and retroviral proteins, *Mol. Cell. Biol.* **5:**1630–1638.

Nishioka, Y., Leder, A., and Leder, P., 1980, Unusual α-globin-like gene that has clearly lost both globin intervening sequences, *Proc. Natl. Acad. Sci. U.S.A.* **77:**2806–2809.

Singh, H., Bieker, J. J., and Dumas, L. B., 1982, Genetic transformation of *Saccharomyces cerevisiae* with single-stranded circular DNA vectors, *Gene* **20:**441–449.

Varmus, H. E., 1983, Retroviruses, in: *Mobile Genetic Elements* (J. A. Shapiro, ed.), Academic Press, New York, pp. 411–503.

Winston, F., Durbin, K. J., and Fink, G. R., 1984a, The *SPT3* gene is required for normal transcription of Ty elements in *Saccharomyces cerevisiae, Cell* **39**(2):675–682.

Winston, F., Chaleff, D. T. L., Valent, B., and Fink, G. R., 1984b, Mutations affecting Ty-mediated expression of the HIS4 gene of *Saccharomyces cerevisiae, Genetics* **107:**179–197.

Woudt, L. P., Pastink, A., Kempers-Veenstra, A. E., Jansen, A. E. M., Mager, W. H., and Planta, R. J., 1983, The genes coding for histone H3 and H4 in *Neurospora crassa* are unique and contain intervening sequences, *Nucleic Acids Res.* **11:**5347–5360.

6

Comparative Genetic Analysis of Homeobox Genes in Mouse and Man

FRANK H. RUDDLE, CHARLES P. HART, MARK RABIN, ANNE FERGUSON-SMITH, and DIMITRINA PRAVTCHEVA

1. Introduction

Homeobox sequences in insects have been described as repetitive elements in homeotic genes (McGinnis *et al.*, 1984a). They have also been found in other genes that have developmental functions. The homeobox sequences are conserved in many animal groups across the protostome and deuterostome lineages of evolutionary ascent. Highly conserved homeobox sequences have been described in numerous vertebrates, including amphibians and mammals (McGinnis *et al.*, 1984b). We have been especially concerned with homeobox sequences in the mouse and in man (McGinnis *et al.*, 1984c). It is now certain that the homeobox sequences code domains within functional genes in vertebrates, on the basis of their expression in polyadenylated RNA transcripts (Hart *et al.*, 1985). Moreover, the tissue-specific expression and temporal patterns of expression are both consistent with a developmental role (Awgulewitsch *et al.*, 1986).

This chapter will compare the map positions of homeobox sequences in man and mouse. We have emphasized genetic linkage relationships in our studies, since map positions provide a way of characterizing individual homeoboxes, determining patterns of clustering, and detecting identity with

FRANK H. RUDDLE, CHARLES P. HART, MARK RABIN, ANNE FERGUSON-SMITH, and DIMITRINA PRAVTCHEVA • Department of Biology, Yale University, New Haven, Connecticut 06511.

or relationship to genes of biological interest (Ruddle *et al.*, 1985a). Since the homeobox linkage information in the mouse *Mus musculus* is more complete, we will discuss this first.

2. Murine Homeobox Genes

If we consider homeobox sequences that show a high degree of sequence homology with the *Drosophila* homeoboxes in the ultrabithorax (*Ubx*) and antennapedia (*Antp*) genes, we recognize three loci, namely, *Hox-1, -2,* and *-3,* that map, respectively, to mouse chromosomes 6, 11, and 15. The high degree of sequence homology within the *Ubx–Antp* family is shown in Fig. 1 (Ruddle *et al.*, 1985b).

The *Hox-1* locus was initially mapped to mouse chromosome 6 by somatic-cell-hybrid mapping (McGinnis *et al.*, 1984c). A similar approach has shown that the locus maps proximal to the *IgK* locus, and recent work in Peter Gruss's laboratory shows that it maps between the β T-cell-receptor locus on chromosome 6 and *IgK* (personal communication). Previous published data and more recent unpublished data taken together indicate that at least six homeobox sequences reside within a distance of approximately 50 kilobases at the *Hox-1* locus on chromosome 6. The individual homeoboxes within this cluster are currently known by trivial names. We recommend that they be numbered serially, i.e., *Hox-1.1, -1.2,* etc. Moreover, in agreement with standard practice in mammalian gene mapping, we believe that species designations should not be incorporated into the formal gene name, but rather that species identification be handled informally and *ad hoc*. One would thus speak of "murine" or "human" forms of *Hox-1.1*. Sufficient data on the physical placement of homeobox sequence within *Hox-1* will soon be sufficiently complete to implement such nomenclature if a majority of workers in this field agree.

A second *Hox* locus, *Hox-2,* has been shown to map to the middle region of mouse chromosome 11 in the vicinity of *Rex* (Hart *et al.*, 1985). This locus also represents a cluster of homeoboxes containing at least six sequences. Four of these sequences have already been named according to the scheme recommended above for *Hox-1* homeoboxes (Fig. 2).

A third homeobox locus in the *Ubx–Antp* family, *Hox-3,* maps to mouse chromosome 15 (Awgulewitsch *et al.*, 1986). Only one homeobox sequence has currently been detected at this locus.

3. Human Homeobox Genes

It is of interest to determine whether human cognates of the mouse homeobox loci exist. We have mapped human loci in two general ways: by using human specific homeobox clones and by using mouse probes to identify their human counterparts. Both methods have provided useful comparative data. Human probes, designated Hu-1 and Hu-2, used in conjunction with the chromosome *in situ* hybridization procedure reveal a human locus at 17q11–22 (Rabin *et al.*, 1985). This locus has subsequently been shown to be homologous with mouse locus *Hox-2*, on the basis of DNA-hybridization and DNA-sequencing studies (Hart *et al.*, 1985; Joyner *et al.*, 1985b). As a result of these comparisons, we have designated the human locus on chromosome 17 as *Hox-2*. The individual homeoboxes have been designated as *Hox-2.1*, *-2.2*, etc., consistent with our recommendations for the naming of murine *Hox-1* (Fig. 2).

A human locus homologous to mouse *Hox-1* has been identified recently in our laboratory by Mark Rabin and Ann Ferguson-Smith, using cross-species *in situ* hybridization in conjunction with mouse *Hox-1* probes (Rabin *et al.*, 1986). This locus, designated human *Hox-1*, maps to the midregion of the short arm of human chromosome 7, at 7p14–p21.

Attempts are currently being made to identify the human genetic cognate of the mouse *Hox-3* locus. As yet, no obvious human counterpart has been located, although a homologous human sequence has been identified by hybridization analysis.

A separate, more distantly homologous family of homeoboxes known as *engrailed* exists in *Drosophila*. A mouse homologue of engrailed has been mapped to mouse chromosome 1 by G. Martin and her collaborators and is designated *En-1* (Joyner *et al.*, 1985a). This locus has been mapped within several centimorgans of the murine morphogenetic locus *Dominant hemimelia*. As yet, no cognate human locus has been reported.

4. Comparative Genetic Relationships between Species

When we compare the chromosomes bearing homeobox sequences, we see patterns of conserved linkage relationships for other genes as well (see Green, 1981; de la Chapelle, 1985). Mouse chromosome 6 and human chromosome 7 show a homologous relationship for the genes T-cell-receptor β-chain (*TCRB*), carboxypeptidase (*CPA*), and trypsin I (*TRY1*)

Block 1 — N-terminal arm (positions −7 to −1)

Protein	−7	−6	−5	−4	−3	−2	−1
Antp	Ile	Tyr	Leu	Glu	Pro	Thr	—
Mo-10	Gly	Pro	Pro	Gly	Gln	Ala	Glu
Hu-1	Ser	Arg	Tyr	Asp	Gly	Pro	Ser
Hu-2	Thr	Gly	Ser	Ser	Phe	Gly	Asp
AC1	Gly	Val	Gly	Tyr	Gly	Ser	Pro
MM3	Leu	Ser	Leu	Ala	Gly	Ala	Asp

(annotations: hpo · Ala · *)

Block 2 — positions 1 to 20

Protein	1	2	3	4	5	6	7	8	9	10	11	12	13	14	15	16	17	18	19	20
Antp	Arg	Lys	Arg	Gly	Arg	Gln	Thr	Tyr	Thr	Arg	Tyr	Gln	Thr	Leu	Glu	Leu	Glu	Lys	Glu	Phe
Mo-10	Ser	Lys	Arg	Gly	Arg	Thr	Thr	Pro	Ala	Arg	Tyr	Gln	Thr	Val	Glu	Leu	Glu	Lys	Gly	Phe
Hu-1	Gly	Lys	Arg	Ala	Arg	Thr	Thr	Tyr	Ala	Arg	Tyr	Gln	Thr	Leu	Glu	Leu	Glu	Lys	Glu	Phe
Hu-2	Thr	Ala	Gly	Gly	Gly	Gln	Thr	Tyr	Thr	Ser	Tyr	Gln	Thr	Leu	Glu	Leu	Glu	Lys	Glu	Phe
AC1	Arg	Arg	Arg	Gly	Arg	Gln	Ser	Tyr	Ile	Arg	Tyr	Gln	Thr	Leu	Glu	Leu	Glu	Lys	Glu	Phe
MM3	Arg	Lys	Arg	Gly	Arg	Gln	Thr	Tyr	Thr	Arg	Tyr	Gln	Thr	Leu	Glu	Leu	Glu	Lys	Glu	Phe

(annotations: hpo · *)

Block 3 — positions 21 to 40 (Helix 2)

Protein	21	22	23	24	25	26	27	28	29	30	31	32	33	34	35	36	37	38	39	40
Antp	His	Phe	Asn	Arg	Tyr	Leu	Thr	Arg	Arg	Arg	Arg	Ile	Glu	Ile	Ala	His	Ala	Leu	Cys	Leu
Mo-10	His	Phe	Asn	Arg	Tyr	Leu	Met	Pro	Arg	Arg	Arg	Val	Glu	Ile	Ala	Met	Ala	Leu	Asn	Leu
Hu-1	His	Phe	Asn	Arg	Tyr	Leu	Thr	Arg	Arg	Arg	Arg	Ile	Glu	Ile	Ala	His	Ala	Leu	Cys	Leu
Hu-2	His	Tyr	Asn	Arg	Tyr	Leu	Thr	Arg	Arg	Arg	Arg	Ile	Glu	Ile	Ala	His	Ala	His	Cys	Leu
AC1	His	Phe	Asn	Arg	Tyr	Leu	Thr	Arg	Arg	Arg	Arg	Ile	Glu	Ile	Ala	Asn	Ala	Leu	Cys	Leu
MM3	His	Phe	Asn	Arg	Tyr	Leu	Thr	Arg	Arg	Arg	Arg	Ile	Glu	Ile	Ala	His	Val	Leu	Cys	Leu

Block 1 — Helix 3 region (positions 41–60). Markers: position 45 = Ile/Val*, position 48 = hpo*.

Gene	41	42	43	44	45*	46	47	48*	49	50	51	52	53	54	55	56	57	58	59	60
Antp	Thr	Glu	Arg	Gln	Ile	Lys	Ile	Trp	Phe	Gln	Asn	Arg	Arg	Met	Lys	Trp	Lys	Lys	Glu	Asn
Mo-10	Thr	Glu	Arg	Gln	Ile	Lys	Ile	Trp	Phe	Gln	Asn	Arg	Arg	Met	Lys	Tyr	Lys	Lys	Asp	Gln
Hu-1	Ser	Glu	Arg	Gln	Ile	Lys	Ile	Trp	Phe	Gln	Asn	Arg	Arg	Met	Lys	Trp	Lys	Lys	Asp	Asn
Hu-2	Thr	Glu	Arg	Gln	Ile	Lys	Ile	Trp	Phe	Gln	Asn	Arg	Arg	Met	Lys	Trp	Lys	Lys	Glu	Ser
AC1	Thr	Glu	Arg	Gln	Ile	Lys	Ile	Trp	Phe	Gln	Asn	Arg	Arg	Met	Lys	Trp	Lys	Lys	Glu	Arg
MM3	Thr	Glu	Arg	Gln	Ile	Lys	Ile	Trp	Phe	Gln	Asn	Arg	Arg	Met	Lys	Trp	Lys	Lys	Glu	Asn

Block 2 — C-terminal region (positions 61–67 and following):

Gene	61	62	63	64	65	66	67		
Antp	Lys	Gly	Gly	Leu	Thr	Ala	Ser	Pro	Gln
Mo-10	Lys	Gly	Gly	Met	Thr	Ala	Ser	Lys	Gln
Hu-1	Leu	Leu	Ser	Met	Leu	Ser	Leu	Ser	Glu
Hu-2	Leu	Leu	Ser	Ala	Leu	Ser	Gln	Leu	Glu
AC1	Asn	Leu	Ser	Thr	Leu	Thr	Leu	Ser	Asn
MM3	Lys	Ala	Ser	Pro	Ser	Pro	Ser	Pro	… Stop

Figure 1. Comparisons of homeobox sequences. *Drosophila* (Antp), mouse (Mo-10), human (Hu-1, Hu-2), and *Xenopus* (AC1, MM3) sequences are shown. Helix 2 and Helix 3 in the 3′ region relate to structural similarities with prokaryotic DNA-binding and -regulating proteins such as λ repressor. Reproduced from Ruddle *et al.* (1985b).

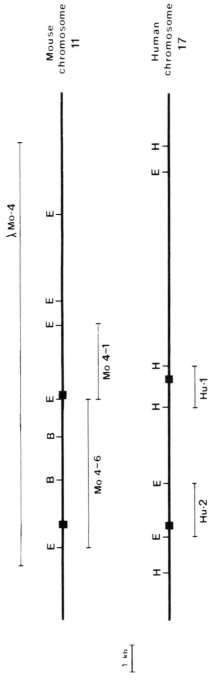

Figure 2. Comparisons of human and mouse homologous regions in *Hox-2*. (■) Homeoboxes. Reproduced from Hart *et al.*, (1985).

(Fig. 3). It should be noted that these genes map to the long arm of chromosome 7 in man, whereas the *Hox-1* locus maps to the short arm, suggesting at least two separated conserved regions between human chromosome 7 and mouse 6. The genes *TRY1* and *CPA* have not yet been regionally mapped.

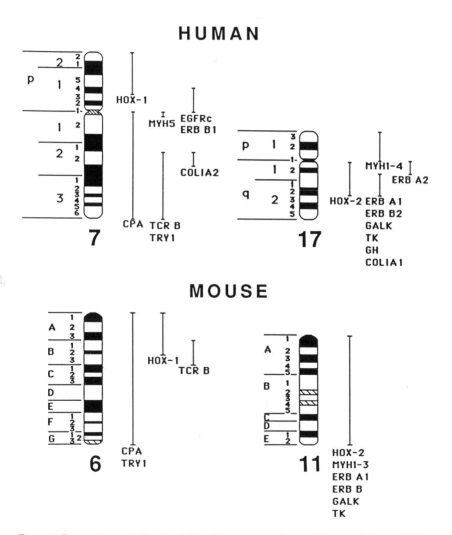

Figure 3. Comparisons of *Hox-1* and *Hox-2* in mouse and man. Gene symbols are defined in the text.

Human chromosome 17 likewise shows a homologous relationship to mouse chromosome 11. The homologous genes in common in this instance are transforming antigen 53 (*TP53*), myosin heavy chains (*MYH*), galactokinase (*GALK*), thymidine kinase (*TK*), avian erythroblastic leukemia viral oncogene homologue A1 (*ERBA1*), avian erythroblastic leukemia viral oncogene homologue B2 (*ERBB2*), collagen type I $\alpha-1$ (*COL1A1*), small nuclear RNA (snRNA), and tissue-specific extinguisher (*TSE*1). Again, more than one region of homology is indicated, since in man this cognate gene set is distributed to both the short and long arms of chromosome 17.

Comparisons for mouse chromosome 15 cannot yet be made, because the human *Hox-3* counterpart has not yet been identified. However, it is known that four human chromosomes, namely, 8, 12, 16, and 22, show genetic homology with mouse chromosome 15. These, then, become candidates for the position of human *Hox-3*.

5. Comparative Genetic Relationships within Species

We see evidence in man of genetic relatedness between the chromosomes that bear homeobox sequences. The epidermal-growth-factor receptor (*EGFR*) that maps to human chromosome 7p has a highly related sequence on human chromosome 17q. This is *ERBB2*, which has been shown in man (chromosome 17) to be a functional second *EGFR* (Yamamoto *et al.*, 1986). Thus, it is likely that there are two *EGFRs*: one on 7, another on 17. These can be referred to, respectively, as *EGFR-1* and *EGFR-2*. In the mouse, an *ERBB* gene has been mapped to mouse chromosome 11. If the mouse follows the human homologies, one would predict a similar sequence on mouse chromosome 6. In man, the *EGFR* genes map in the same vicinities as homeobox loci *Hox-1* and *-2*. It will be of interest to determine whether a similar proximal pattern of linkage obtains in the mouse as well. It should also be noted that in man, the *COL1A2* gene maps to chromosome 7, whereas the *COL1A1* maps to 17, again underscoring a genetic relatedness between these two chromosomes.

In the mouse, the *Int1* gene maps to mouse chromosome 15 in the vicinity of *Hox-3*. The function or functions of the *Int* genes are unknown, although they code for transcripts that are expressed with temporal and tissue specificity (Moore *et al.*, 1986; Casey *et al.*, 1986). They have been revealed by the integration of mammary tumor viruses in their vicinity with consequent effects on their expression. In man, *Int-1* maps to 12pter–q14. This recommends chromosome 12 as a candidate for human *Hox-3*.

A possibly interesting relationship involves the mouse gene little (*lit*), which maps near murine *Hox-1* on mouse chromosome 6, and the human growth hormone (*GH*) gene that maps close to human *Hox-2* on human chromosome 17. The *lit* mutation results in dwarf mice as a consequence of growth-hormone deficiency. This has recently been reported to be the result of a defective interaction between the growth-hormone-releasing factor and its receptor (Jansson *et al.*, 1986). It will be of interest to determine, possibly by sequence analysis, whether there is a similarity between the growth-hormone and the growth-hormone-releasing systems that can be explained in terms of an evolutionary relationship.

6. Possible Functional Relationships between Homeobox Loci and Linked Genes

6.1. Mouse Hox-1, Chromosome 6

As stated above, *Hox-1* has been mapped to an interval between *TCRB* and the immunoglobulin kappa (*IgK*) locus. The *lit* gene discussed above maps to this region. A gene that controls a zona pellucida protein has recently been mapped to mouse chromosome 6, but its subregional position is not known (P. Lalley, personal communication). Morphogenetic mutants that could bear a relationship to *Hox-1* are hypodactyly (*Hd*) and hydrocephalic–polydactyl (*hpy*). We are currently establishing the genetic order of and distances between these genetic markers and *Hox-1*.

6.2. Mouse Hox-2, Chromosome 11

The *ERBB2* gene has already been discussed. Recently in collaboration with Dr. Corden of Johns Hopkins University, we mapped the RNA polymerase II large-subunit gene by *in situ* hybridization to chromosome II (Pravtcheva *et al.*, 1986). The *Drosophila* homologue of this gene maps to the *Drosophila* X chromosome, and a mutant form has been described as a *Ubx-like* allele, because it mimicked the action of the homeotic gene. More recently, its *Ubx* action has been interpreted as a nonspecific effect induced by the altered form of the mutated polymerase. However, murine linkage relationship suggests a more direct relationship that should be examined further. The *U1A1* snRNA locus has recently been mapped to a position close to *Re* (Michael *et al.*, 1986). It is of interest that the human *U2* snRNA locus maps near the *Hox-2* locus on human chromosome 17. A number of mutant genes have been reported in the region of *Hox-2* that affect hair development (*Re, lt, Al*), the central nervous system (*shm*), and the skeleton (*Ts*). These are rex (*Re*), lustrous (*lt*), and alopecia (*Al*); shambling (*shm*); and tail short (*Ts*).

6.3. Mouse Hox-3, Chromosome 15

Two protooncogenes, *c-myc* and *c-sis*, have been shown to map at the distal end of chromosome 15 in the vicinity of *Hox-3* (Somssich *et al.*, 1984). As discussed above, *Int-1* also maps in this region (H. Hameister, personal communication). In addition to these genes, a series of mutations that affect hair development (*hl, Sha, Ca, N*), the nervous system (*sw, med*), skeletal development (*Ht*), ectodermal differentiation (*Ve*), and possibly iron transport (*mk*) have been mapped to this region. These are hair loss (*hl*), shaven (*Sha*), caracul (*Ca*), and naked (*N*); swaying (*sw*) and motor endplate disease (*med*); high tail (*Ht*); velvet coat (*Ve*); and microcytic anemia (*mk*). It is interesting that genes having somewhat similar properties are in linkage with mouse *Hox-2* and *-3*, these being the neurological mutants shambling (*shm*, chromosome 11) vs. swaying (*sw*, chromosome 15) and rex (*Re*, chromosome 11) vs. caracul (Ca, chromosome 15).

6.4. Human Hox-1, Chromosome 7

Hox-1 has recently been mapped to the midregion of the short arm. Genes of interest with respect to growth and differentiation in this region are the T-cell-receptor γ-chain (*TCRG*) and the epidermal-growth-factor receptor (*EGFR*). Other genes of possible interest, but at a distance from *Hox-1* or as yet unmapped, are the histone genes (H1, H2A, H2B, H3F1, H4F1), T-cell receptor β-chain (*TCRB*), collagen 1α2 (*COL1A2*), myosin heavy chain 5 (*MYH5*), and growth control factor 1 (*GCF1*).

6.5. Human Hox-2, Chromosome 17

Human *Hox-2* maps to 17q11–22. There are numerous genes with a relationship to cellular growth and differentiation that map to this region. They are collagen type 1α1 (*COL1A1*), one of the ubiquitous and early, developmentally expressed collagens; *ERBB2*, in all likelihood a second *EGFR*, as indicated above; *ERBA*, which was recently shown to be related to the estrogen-type peptide receptors that have DNA-binding and gene-regulatory properties (Chambon *et al.*, 1986); the growth hormone–placental lactogen complex; gastrin (*GAS*), a peptide hormone with homology to growth hormone that is expressed not only in the digestive tract, but also in the central nervous system (Rehfeld, 1981); the nerve-growth-factor receptor (*NGFR*) (Huebner *et al.*, 1986); thymidine kinase (*TK*); the U2 snRNA cluster (*RNVZ*); and the crystallin β-polypeptide 1 (*CRYB1*). We have previously noted that additional genes of interest, such as transforming protein 53 (*TP53*) and myosin heavy chains 1–4 (MYH1–4), map to other more distant sites on chromosome 17. The tissue-specific extinguisher (*TSE-1*) gene that inhibits hepatocyte-specific expression and has the properties of a transacting, regulatory protein also maps to chromosome 17; however, its regional localization has not yet been defined (Killary and Fournier, 1984; Petit *et al.*, 1986).

7. Discussion

The homeobox system represents a homologous family of sequences present in broadly divergent animal forms. The number of sequences is small and generally comparable in different species. In *Drosophila*, mouse, and man, there is evidence for clustering into gene complexes. These clusters span distances approximately 5- to 6-fold shorter in mammals than in *Drosophila*. The presence of multiple copies of the homeobox sequences in divergent forms suggests that the family may have arisen through gene duplications at an early time in evolution.

Evidence exists that the homeobox sequences specify a DNA-binding domain. This comes from comparisons of homeobox structure and sequence and from direct experimentation. Deduced amino acid sequence analysis of homeoboxes has revealed a structural similarity to prokaryotic trans-regulatory binding proteins, such as the lac repressor and the λ repressor (Laughon and Scott, 1984). Direct sequence homology also exists with elements of the yeast mating-type system, which are known to function as DNA-regulatory proteins (Shepherd *et al.*, 1984). Experiments dealing with *Drosophila* homeotic gene products have shown that fusion proteins of polypeptides containing homeoboxes have the capacity to bind DNA (Desplan *et al.*, 1985). Recently, we have carried out similar studies in the mouse, directly demonstrating a DNA-binding property of homeobox-coded products (A. Fainsod and L. Bogarad, unpublished data).

If, as we suggest, the homeobox genetic elements have multiplied by DNA duplications, and if, as we believe, the products of the genes are DNA-binding and -regulating, then it follows that the sum of these elements may function as a coordinated whole. Adaptive changes in the system would permit the detection of defined combinations of environmental signals that would then be translated into a defined and limited set of expressions. A portion of the output could be thought of as cybernetic, serving to stabilize or alter expression, while a portion would be directed to the hierarchical control of genes necessary for growth, differentiation, and morphogenesis. Lewis (1985) has put forward a similar model based on the bithorax complex of many years ago, which has recently been revised.

We believe that this hypothesis is a useful way to view the homeobox gene system, because it offers testable predictions. It suggests that genes involved in the homeobox network may tend to be physically proximal to the homeobox genes. It also suggests that they may possess homologous sequences. Thus, it will be of interest in the future to examine the high-resolution linkage relationships of genes surrounding the homeobox genes. We believe this may be especially productive in the case of human *Hox-2* on human chromosome 17, since so many genes having a possible role in growth and differentiation are located in this region. In addition to studying linkage order and distance, it will also be of interest to compare the base-pair sequences in the coding and noncoding regions of these neighboring genes.

References

Awgulewitsch, A., Utset, M. F., Hart, C. P., McGinnis, W., and Ruddle, F. H., 1986, Spatial restriction in expression of a mouse homeobox locus within the central nervous system, *Nature (London)* **320:**328–335.

Casey, G., Smith, R., McGillivray, D., Peters, G., and Dickson, C., 1986, Characterization and chromosome assignment of the human homolog of int-2, a potential proto-oncogene, *Mol. Cell. Biol.* **6:**502–510.

Chambon, P., Green, S., Walter, P., Kumar, V., Krust, A., Bornert, J., and Bonner, D., 1986, Steroid hormone receptor genes: Cloning, organization, and expression, *ISCU Newsletter* **4:**246–249.

De la Chapelle, A., 1985, Human gene mapping 8, *Cytogenet. Cell Genet.* **40**(1–4):1–823.

Desplan, C., Theis, J., and O'Farrell, P., 1985, The *Drosophila* developmental gene, engrailed, encodes a sequence-specific DNA binding activity, *Nature (London)* **318**:630–635.

Green, M. C., 1981, *Genetic Variants and Strains of the Laboratory Mouse*, Gustav Fischer Verlag, Stuttgart .

Hart, C. P., Awgulewitsch, F., Fainsod, A., McGinnis, W., and Ruddle, F. H., 1985, Homeo-box gene complex on mouse chromosome 11: Molecular cloning, expression in embryogenesis and homology to a human homeo-box locus, *Cell* **43**:9–18.

Huebner, K., Isobe, M., Chao, M., Bothwell, M., Ross, A., Finan, J., Hoxie, J., Seghal, A., Buck, C. R., Lanahan, A., Nowell, P., Koprowski, H., and Croce, C., 1986, The nerve growth factor receptor gene is at human chromosome region 17q12–17q22, distal to the chromosome 17 breakpoint in acute leukemias, *Proc. Natl. Acad. Sci. U.S.A.* **83**:1403–1407.

Jansson, J.-O., Downs, T., Beamer, W., and Frohman, L., 1986, Receptor-association resistance to growth hormone-releasing factor in dwarf "little" mice, *Science* **232**:511–512.

Joyner, A. L., Kornberg, T., Coleman, K. G., Cox, D. R., and Martin, G. R., 1985a, Expression during embryogenesis of a mouse gene with sequence homology to the *Drosophila engrailed* gene, *Cell* **43**:29–37.

Joyner, A. L., Hauser, C., Kornberg, T., Tjian, R., and Martin, G., 1985b, Structure and expression of two classes of Mammalian homeo-box-containing genes, *Cold Spring Harbor Symp. Quant. Biol.* **50**:291–300.

Killary, A., and Fournier, R., 1984, A genetic analysis of extinction: *Trans*-dominant loci regulate expression of liver-specific traits in hepatoma hybrid cells, *Cell* **38**:523–534.

Laughon, A., and Scott, M. P., 1984, Sequence of a *Drosophila* segmentation gene: Protein structure homology with DNA binding proteins, *Nature (London)* **310**:25–31.

Lewis, E. B., 1985, Regulation of the genes of the bithorax complex in *Drosophila*, in: *Banbury Report 20: Genetic Manipulations of the Early mammalian Embryos* (F. Costantini and R. Jaenisch, eds.), Cold Spring Harbor Laboratory, Cold Spring Harbor, New York, pp. 155–164.

McGinnis, W., Levine, M., Hafen, E., Kuroiwa, A., and Gehring, W. J., 1984a, A conserved DNA sequence in homeotic genes of the *Drosophila* antennapedia and bithorax complexes, *Nature (London)* **308**:428–433.

McGinnis, W., Garber, R. L., Witz, J., Kuroiwa, A., and Gehring, W. J., 1984b, A homologous protein-coding sequence in *Drosophila* homeotic genes and its conservation to other metazoans, *Cell* **37**:408–412.

McGinnis, W., Hart, C. P., Gehring, W. J., and Ruddle, F. H., 1984c, Molecular cloning and chromosome mapping of a mouse DNA sequence homologous to homeotic genes of *Drosophila*, *Cell* **38**:675–680.

Michael, S. K., Hilger, J., Kozak, C., Whitney, J. B. III, and Howard, E. F., 1986, Characterization and mapping of DNA sequence homologous to mouse Ula1 snRNA: Localization on chromosome 11 near the *Dlb-1* and *Re* loci, *Somat. Cell Mol. Genet.* **12**(3):215–223.

Moore, R., Casey, G., Brookes, S., Dixon, M., Peters, G., and Dickson, C., 1986, Sequence, topography and protein coding potential of mouse int-2: A putative oncogene activated by mouse mammary tumor virus, *Eur. Mol. Biol. Org. J.* **5**:919–924.

Petit, C., Levilliers, J., Ott, M.-O., and Weiss, M., 1986, Tissue-specific expression of the rat albumin gene: Genetic control of its extinction in microcell hybrids, *Proc. Natl. Acad. Sci. U.S.A.* **83**:2561–2565.

Pravtcheva, D., Rabin, M., Bartolomei, M., Gorden, J., and Ruddle, F. H., 1986, Chromosomal assignment of the gene encoding the largest subunit of RNA polymerase II in the mouse, *Somat. All. Mol. Genet.* (in press).

Rabin, M., Hart, C. P., Ferguson-Smith, A., McGinnis, W., Levine, M., and Ruddle, F. H., 1985, Two homeobox loci mapped in evolutionarily related mouse human chromosomes, *Nature (London)* **314**:175–178.

Rabin, M., Ferguson-Smith, A., Hart, C.P., and Ruddle, F. H., 1986, Cognate homeobox loci mapped on homologous human and mouse chromosomes, *Proc. Natl. Acad. Sci. U.S.A.* (in press).

Rehfeld, J. F., 1981, Four basic characteristics of the gastrin–cholecystokinin system, *Am. J. Physiol.* **240**:G255–G266.

Ruddle, F. H., Hart, C. P., Awgulewitsch, A., Fainsod, A., Utset, M., Dalton, D., Kerk, N., Rabin, M., Ferguson-Smith, A., Fienberg, A., and McGinnis, W., 1985a, Mammalian homeo box genes, *Cold Spring Harbor Symp. Quant. Biol.* **50**:277–284.

Ruddle, F. H., Hart, C. P., and McGinnis, W., 1985b, Homeo-box sequences—relevant vertebrate developmental mechanisms, *Banbury Report 20: Genetic Manipulations of the Early Mammalian Embryo* (F. Costantini and R. Jaenisch, eds.), Cold Spring Harbor Laboratory, Cold Spring Harbor, New York, pp. 169–177.

Shepherd, J. C. W., McGinnis, W., Carrasco, A. E., DeRobertis, E. M., and Gehring, W. J., 1984, Fly and frog homeo domains show homologies with yeast mating type regulatory proteins, *Nature (London)* **310**:70–72.

Somssich, I., Spira, J., Hameister, H., and Klein, G., 1984, Correlation between tumorigenicity and banding patterns of chromosome 15 in murine T-cell leukemia cells and hybrids of normal and malignant cells, *Chromosoma* **91**:39–45.

Yamamoto, T., Ikawa, S., Akiyama, T., Semba, K., Nomura, N., Miyajima, N., Saito, T., and Toyoshima, K., 1986, Similarity of protein encoded by the human c-erb-B-2 gene to epidermal growth factor receptor, *Nature (London)* **319**:230–231.

7

Eukaryotic Transcriptional Specificity Conferred by DNA-Binding Proteins

JAMES T. KADONAGA, MICHAEL R. BRIGGS,
and ROBERT TJIAN

1. Introduction

The pattern of gene expression in mammalian cells requires thousands of genes to be turned on and off in a temporally and spatially regulated manner. The control of transcription initiation is one means by which expression of genes can be varied. Regulation of transcription initiation is well characterized in prokaryotes, but in higher organisms such as humans, this phenomenon is only beginning to be clarified. One common approach to this problem has been the identification of important *cis*-acting DNA sequences in the region surrounding transcription initiation sites.

The principal method of identifying the DNA sequence elements that control transcription in eukaryotes has been to mutagenize DNA sequences near the start site of transcription and then to test the altered templates, either by reintroduction into the cell or by introduction into experimental substitutes such as an *in vitro* transcription system. Accumulation of new RNA or protein is measured, and the effect of sequence alterations on the promoter strength is thus revealed. These studies have shown that promoters for protein-coding genes vary in sequence, yet are organized according to a common plan.

Many promoters have an AT-rich element called a TATA box, which is located 25–30 base pairs (bp) upstream from the beginning of the tran-

JAMES T. KADONAGA, MICHAEL R. BRIGGS, and ROBERT TJIAN • Department of Biochemistry, University of California, Berkeley, California 94720.

scribed sequence. Mutation of this region generates 5' heterogeneity in the transcripts, although the overall level of RNA synthesis may not be significantly reduced (Ghosh *et al.*, 1981; Benoist and Chambon, 1980). Further upstream from the start site of transcription is a region containing one or more additional promoter elements. Some upstream elements, such as the GC box, have now been found in many different promoters (Myers *et al.*, 1981; Fromm and Berg, 1982; Everett *et al.*, 1983; Kadonaga *et al.*, 1986), while others such as the metallothionein metal regulatory element (Stuart *et al.*, 1984) and the heat-shock regulatory element (Pelham, 1982), appear to have a more restricted function.

The activity of many promoters is also influenced by an enhancer, which is a separate regulatory element (Banerji *et al.*, 1981; Fromm and Berg, 1982; Moreau *et al.*, 1981). The enhancer can be 1000 bp or more from the promoter and may be located either upstream or downstream from the transcription start site. The prototype enhancer has been found in simian virus 40 (SV40), but control elements with similar properties have also been found in other viruses and in the cellular genome. Some enhancers appear to be tissue-specific (Queen and Baltimore, 1983; Picard and Shaffner, 1984), whereas others mediate transcriptional responses of genes to steroid hormones (Chandler *et al.*, 1983).

The understanding of promoter function gained by the analysis of DNA sequences has certain limitations that could be overcome by the identification, purification, and characterization of proteins required for transcription. The enzyme responsible for messenger RNA (mRNA) synthesis, RNA polymerase II, differs from prokaryotic RNA holoenzyme in that it seems to lack any inherent ability to recognize promoters in an *in vitro* reaction. It has recently become clear that crude extracts from eukaryotic cells contain factors that impart promoter specificity to the purified RNA polymerase II and allow *in vitro* initiation of transcription at the same start sites used *in vivo* (Weil *et al.*, 1979; Dynan and Tjian, 1981). Some of these factors seem to be required for initiation at all promoters, whereas others are required for initiation at a subset of all promoters (Dynan and Tjian, 1983a). Many of the promoter-specific factors are sequence-specific DNA-binding proteins (Dynan and Tjian, 1983b, 1985; Jones *et al.*, 1985; Parker and Topol, 1984; Sawadogo and Roeder, 1985). In the ideal situation, the binding activities and transcriptional properties of a factor have been related experimentally with sequence-specific binding- and transcription-stimulatory activities copurifying during fractionation.

2. Results and Discussion

2.1. Cis and Trans Regulatory Components of the Simian Virus 40 Promoter

We have used DNA tumor viruses such as SV40 to investigate the mechanisms of transcriptional regulation in animal cells because they provide a relatively simple and valuable model for studying transcriptional specificity. Important *cis* regulatory elements of the SV40 early promoter have been mapped, and reconstituted *in vitro* transcription reactions have allowed us to identify and isolate specific cellular factors that recognize and bind to the viral promoter. Analyses of the viral promoter mutants both *in vivo* and *in vitro* have established that a region of approximately 300 bp adjacent to the origin of DNA replication contains multiple *cis* regulatory elements responsible for directing transcription of both early and late viral mRNA synthesis. Mutational analysis of the viral transcription-control region has revealed that the major early promoter consists of three 21-bp repeated elements preceded by a stretch of AT-rich sequences (Fig. 1A) (Myers *et al.*, 1981; Fromm and Berg, 1982; Everett *et al.*, 1983). Early transcription has been shown to initiate predominantly from distinct sites located 20–30 nucleotides downstream from the AT-rich region. In addition, enhancer elements that stimulate early SV40 transcription *in vivo* are located within the 72-bp repeated sequences, which lie 110–250 bp upstream from the early-transcription start sites (Banerji *et al.*, 1981; Fromm and Berg, 1982). Late viral transcription is under the direction of multiple regulatory elements and exhibits a heterogeneous population of start sites scattered throughout the control region. The major initiation site is at nucleotide 325, and several minor ones are located at various adjacent positions (Brady *et al.*, 1982; Hansen and Sharp, 1983; Rio and Tjian, 1984). Transcriptional analysis of various plasmid templates containing the 21-bp repeats in an inverted orientation relative to the AT-rich TATA homology indicates that this upstream promoter sequence can potentiate transcription in a bidirectional manner (Everett *et al.*, 1983; Gidoni *et al.*, 1985).

To dissect the relationship between these various *cis*-acting regulatory sequences and the components of the cellular transcription apparatus that must recognize and interact with them, we have identified the protein factors responsible for activating SV40 RNA synthesis in a cell-free

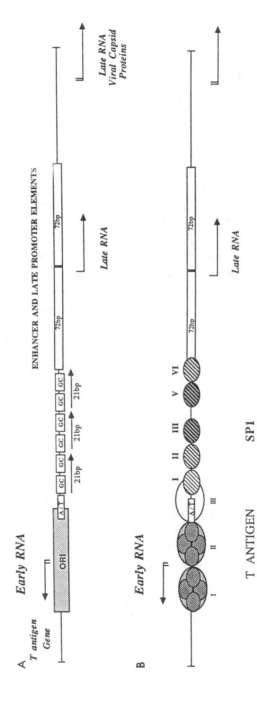

Figure 1. SV40 control region. (A) The diagram depicts various *cis* control sequences represented schematically by rectangular boxes. The large stippled box represents sequences encompassing the SV40 origin of DNA replication. The small open rectangles designate the AT-rich TATA-like element and the six GC-box elements (I, II, III, IV, V, and VI) of the SV40 early promoter. The 21-bp repeats containing the GC-box motifs are underscored by horizontal arrows. The two extended open boxes represent repeated sequences of the 72-bp enhancer elements. The direction of early and late mRNA transcription is designated by arrows pointing left and right, respectively. (B) The dark hatched ellipses represent protomers of the transcription factor Sp1. The large stippled ellipses represent tetramers of T antigen sequentially bound to its recognition sites that overlap the origin of DNA replication.

transcription reaction (Dynan and Tjian, 1983a, b; Gidoni *et al.*, 1984, 1985). Fractionation of HeLa-cell extracts resulted in the identification of a transcription factor, Sp1, that binds selectively to the hexanucleotide sequence, GGGCGG (GC box), that is tandemly repeated six times in the 21-bp elements of SV40 (Fig. 1B). The presence of Sp1 in reconstituted *in vitro* transcription reaction enhances RNA synthesis by RNA polymerase II 10- to 50-fold from a select group of promoters that contain at least one properly positioned GC box. There appear to be approximately 50,000 Sp1 molecules per cell, and the protein has recently been purified 50,000-fold to an estimated 95% homogeneity (Briggs, *et al.*, 1986; Kadonaga and Tjian, 1986). The estimated molecular weight of Sp1 by sodium dodecylsulfate–polyacrylamide gel electrophoresis is 105,000.

The most direct and specific assay of Sp1 activity is deoxyribonuclease (DNase)I or dimethylsulfate (DMS) footprinting, in which a ^{32}P-labeled DNA probe that contains at least one Sp1 binding site is incubated with the factor, lightly treated with DNase or DMS, and analyzed by electrophoresis on a denaturing polyacrylamide gel. Regions of DNA that are bound by Sp1 appear as protected areas (Fig. 2). Alternatively, the transcriptional enhancer activity of Sp1 can be measured *in vitro* by reconstituted transcription reactions carried out in the presence or absence of Sp1. A convenient and specific assay for measuring transcription is the primer extension assay (Lebowitz and Ghosh, 1982), whereby a ^{32}P-labeled oligonucleotide that is complementary to a portion of the newly synthesized RNA is hybridized to the transcripts and a complementary DNA (cDNA) strand is synthesized with reverse transcriptase and subsequently analyzed by electrophoresis on a denaturing polyacrylamide gel (Fig. 2).

The activation of transcription by Sp1 is estimated by comparing the amounts of ^{32}P-labeled cDNA derived from RNA synthesized in the presence and the absence of Sp1. In the SV40 21-bp repeat elements, Sp1–DNA contacts detected by DMS protection fall within a 6-fold repeated sequence moiety of the GC boxes. Sp1 forms strong contacts with five of these GC boxes by interacting with a cluster of guanines within each of these recognition elements. Contacts have so far been detected only in the major groove of the DNA in SV40 and only on one strand (Gidoni *et al.*, 1984). Alteration of individual GC boxes by oligonucleotide-directed mutagenesis suggests the presence of five independently bound protomers within the overall region, with each Sp1 protomer contacting one GC box and protecting approximately 18–20 bp of sequence (Fig. 1B) (Gidoni *et al.*, 1985). This spatial arrangement of Sp1 binding sites sug-

James T. Kadonaga et al.

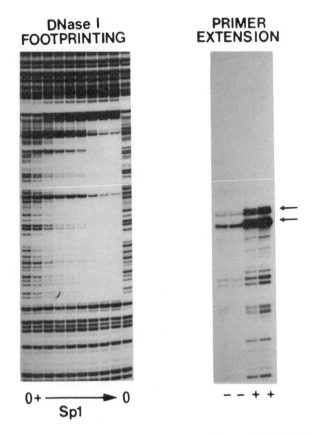

Figure 2. DNase I FOOTPRINTING: The binding of Sp1 to SV40 GC boxes I–VI is depicted, and the footprint boundary is indicated by a bracket. The lanes labeled "0" are negative controls that show the DNase I digestion pattern in the absence of Sp1. In a typical footprint experiment, 5–50 fmoles of ^{32}P-labeled DNA is incubated with 50–500 fmoles of Sp1 monomers before digestion with DNase I. PRIMER EXTENSION: (+) Presence or (−) absence of Sp1. (←) Complementary DNA strands that derive from RNA transcripts generated *in vitro*.

gests that all the bound molecules embrace the DNA from the same face of the molecule and that the five Sp1 protomers are closely aligned on one face of the DNA.

2.2. Role of Sp1 in Other Viral and Cellular Promoters

When Sp1 was first isolated, its interaction with SV40 was thought to be unique. Recently, however, Sp1 has been shown to be required for *in vitro* transcription of several genes, including those of herpes simplex virus (HSV) I (Fig. 3) (Jones *et al.*, 1985; Jones and Tjian, 1985). Both the immediate-early gene *3* and the delayed-early gene *TK* of HSV appear to be Sp1-responsive. The pattern of Sp1-binding sites differs from that of SV40, as each control region in the herpes virus contains multiple separate unit sites of Sp1. Each unit site covers approximately 20 bp and presumably accommodates a single Sp1 protomer. Binding at the TK promoter is particularly interesting because Sp1 appears to interact with distal elements previously defined by mutational analysis (Fig. 4). Moreover, activation is thought to require both Sp1 and a second transcription factor called CAAT-binding transcription factor (CTF), which recognizes and binds in the region between the two Sp1 sites that contain the sequence motif, GCCAAT (Fig. 4) (Jones *et al.*, 1985).

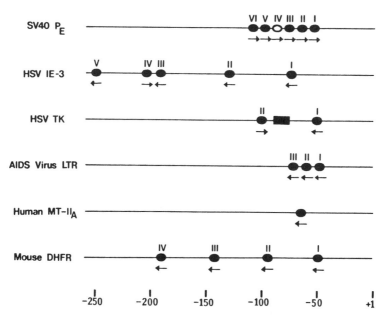

Figure 3. Arrangement of SP1 binding sites in various promoters. Promoters were determined to be Sp1-responsive by *in vitro* transcription in the presence or absence of Sp1. (●) Sp1 binding sites that were characterized by footprinting with Sp1; (▬) binding site for transcription factor CTF, which binds to CCAAT sequences (CAAT boxes). SV40 GC box IV is shown as an open oval because Sp1 bound to GC box V appears to prevent binding of the factor to GC box IV (Gidoni *et al.*, 1985). The orientation of each Sp1 recognition site is indicated by an arrow (NGGGCGGNNN = ←). The RNA start sites are designated +1.

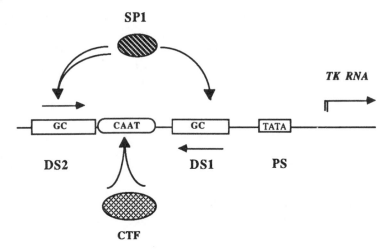

Figure 4. Promoter elements of the HSV *tk* gene. The line diagram depicts multiple *cis* control elements of the *tk* gene consisting of a proximal signal (PS), distal signal 1 (DS1) and distal signal 2 (DS2) represented either as open rectangles (TATA box and GC boxes) or an open ellipse (CAAT box). The inverted GC-box motifs are also designated by horizontal arrows pointing at each other. The direction of transcription is designated by the arrow pointing to the right. The dark hatched ellipse represents a protomer of Sp1. Thick and thin curved arrows emanating from Sp1 designate strong and weak binding to the GC-box motifs of DS2 and DS1, respectively. The cross-hatched large ellipse represents a protomer of CTF bound to the CAAT motif of DS2.

In addition to these viral genes, several cellular sequences also interact with Sp1 (see Fig. 3). A DNA segment of the monkey genome that functions *in vivo* as a bidirectional promoter element contains two Sp1-binding sites (Dynan *et al.*, 1985). Multiple Sp1-binding sites are also found in 5′ flanking sequences of the mouse dihydrofolate reductase gene (Dynan *et al.*, 1986), and multiple or single strong Sp1-binding sites have been identified in human metallothionein I_A and II $_A$ (W. Lee, M. Karin, and R. Tjian, unpublished data). The monkey promoter binding region is relatively large and may be a complex binding site like that of SV40. The mouse dihydrofolate reductase promoter and the metallothionein promoters, by contrast, show unit binding sites similar to those found in herpes virus promoters. Sp1-binding regions usually contain one or more perfect copies of the GC-box hexanucleotide GGGCGG, which may be present in either orientation with respect to transcription. Not all GC boxes bind Sp1 equally well, and sequences outside the core hexanucleotide seem to play an important role in determining the efficiency of binding.

2.3. A Consensus Sp1 Recognition Sequence

Because the GC-box sequence or its inverted form was present in all the Sp1-responsive promoters that were first identified, it was inferred that this hexanucleotide is the recognition sequence for Sp1. However, additional studies have revealed that the GC-box hexanucleotide does not always specify a strong Sp1-binding site and that the decanucleotide consensus sequence shown at the top of Fig. 5 may be a more accurate representation of the recognition sequence (Kadonaga *et al.*, 1986). Except for the 5' G or T, which appear to be equivalent, the upper bases are preferred to the lower ones. Thus, the best Sp1-binding sequences are probably G_4CG_4C and TG_3CG_4C. Interestingly, weak Sp1-binding sites such as the HSV-TK box I and SV40 box I have been found to be important for transcriptional activation (Gidoni *et al.*, 1985; Jones *et al.*, 1985). Thus, in addition to the inherent affinity of the protein for its recognition site, other considerations such as the position of the binding sites relative to the RNA start sites and perhaps direct interaction with other factors, such as CTF- and TATA-binding factors, may be important for Sp1 activation of transcription.

As mentioned previously, a second distinct transcription factor, CTF, appears to act in conjunction with Sp1 to activate transcription from the HSV-TK promoter (see Fig. 4). If this is true, transcription from the TK promoter could be modulated by varying the cellular concentrations of both Sp1 and CTF. Preliminary studies of the metallothionein and β-globin promoters suggest that there may be other sequence-specific DNA-binding proteins that recognize distinct promoter elements and behave like Sp1 and CTF to potentiate transcription (K. A. Jones, J. T. Kadonaga, and R. Tjian, unpublished results). These findings support the hypothesis that there is a class of DNA-binding proteins that can act either alone or in combination with other factors to modulate transcription from a wide range of promoters.

3. Concluding Remarks

Although many details remain to be elucidated, recent work clearly indicates the existence of promoter-specific transcription factors that recog-

$$5'\,{}^{G}_{T}GGGCGG{}^{GGC}_{AAT}3'$$

Sequence	Relative Affinity	Source
G G G G C G G G G C	HIGH	HSV IE-3 (V); DHFR (I,III); MT IIA; CH-TK INTRON; Ha-RAS (I,III,IV)
T G G G C G G G G C	HIGH	HSV IE-3 (III,IV)
T G G G C G G A G T	HIGH	SV40 (III,V)
G G G G C G G A G C	HIGH	DHFR (II,IV)
G A G G C G T G G C	HIGH	AIDS LTR (III)
G G G G C G G G G G	MEDIUM	HSV IE-3 (I); Ha-RAS (II)
G G G G C G G G G T	MEDIUM	HSV IE-3 (II)
C G G G C G G G G C	MEDIUM	Ha-RAS (V)
G A G G C G G A G C	MEDIUM	Ha-RAS (VI)
T G G G C G G G G T	MEDIUM	HSV-TK (II)
T G G G C G G A A C	MEDIUM	SV40 (II)
G G G G C G G G A T	MEDIUM	SV40 (IV)
G G G G C G G G A C	MEDIUM	SV40 (VI)
T G G G C G G G A C	MEDIUM	AIDS LTR (I)
G G G G A G T G G C	MEDIUM	AIDS LTR (II)
G G G G C G G A G A	LOW	SV40 (I)
G G G G C G G C G C	LOW	HSV-TK (I)

Figure 5. A tentative consensus sequence for Sp1 binding. This sequence was derived from the binding sites listed. The relative affinity of Sp1 for each site was estimated by DNase footprinting and is given as HIGH, MEDIUM, or LOW.

nize distinct sequence elements found upstream from the initiation sites in eukaryotic protein-coding genes. Several such factors have now been isolated, and each factor recognizes a different sequence element. Interestingly, there are often multiple binding sites for the same or different factors within a single promoter. Future studies should reveal the role of these protomer-specific transcription factors in the regulation of gene expression in higher organisms.

ACKNOWLEDGMENTS. We thank Kathy Jones, David Gidoni, and Bill Dynan for making major contributions that have allowed many of the conclusions derived herein. This work was supported by grants from the NIH to R.T., and partial support was obtained from an NIEHS center grant. J.T.K. is a Fellow of the Miller Institute.

References

Banerji, J., Rusconi, S., and Schaffner, W., 1981, Expression of a β-globin gene is enhanced by remote SV40 DNA sequences, *Cell* **27**:299–308.

Benoist, C., and Chambon, P., 1980, Deletions covering the putative promoter region of early mRNAs of SV40 do not abolish T antigen expression, *Proc. Natl. Acad. Sci. U.S.A.* **77**:3865–3869.

Brady, J., Radonovich, M., Vodkin, M., Natarajan, V., Thoren, M., Das, G., Janik, J., and Salzman, N. P., 1982, Site-specific base substitution and deletion mutations that enhance or suppress transcription of the SV40 major late RNA, *Cell* **31**:625–633.

Briggs, M. R., Kadonaga, J. T., Bell, S. P., and Tjian, R., 1986, Purification and biochemical characterization of the promoter-specific transcription factor Sp1, *Science* (in press).

Chandler, V. L., Maler, B. A., and Yamamoto, K. R., 1983, DNA sequences bound specifically by glucocorticoid receptor *in vitro* render a heterologous promoter hormone responsive *in vivo*, *Cell* **33**:489–499.

Dynan, W. S., and Tjian, R., 1981, Characterization of factors that impart selectivity to RNA polymerase II in a reconstituted system, in: *Developmental Biology using Purified Genes*, ICN–UCLA Symposium on Molecular and Cellular Biology, Academic Press, New York, pp. 401–414.

Dynan, W. S., and Tjian, R., 1983a, Isolation of transcription factors that discriminate between different promoters recognized by RNA polymerase II, *Cell* **32**:669–680.

Dynan, W. S., and Tjian, R., 1983b, The protomer-specific transcription factor Sp1 binds to upstream sequences in the SV40 early promoter, *Cell* **35**:79–87.

Dynan, W. S., and Tjian, R., 1985, Control of eukaryotic messenger RNA synthesis by sequence-specific DNA binding proteins, *Nature (London)* **316**:774–778.

Dynan, W. S., Saffer, J. D., Lee, W. S., and Tjian, R., 1985, Transcription factor Sp1 recognizes promoter sequences from the monkey genome that are similar to the simian virus 40 promoter, *Proc. Natl. Acad. Sci. U.S.A.* **82**:4915–4919.

Dynan, W. S., Sazer, S., Tjian, R., and Schimke, R. T., 1986, The transcription factor Sp1 recognizes a DNA sequence in the mouse dihydrofolate reductase promoter, *Nature (London)* **319**:246–248.

Everett, R. D., Baty, D., and Chambon, P., 1983, The repeated GC-rich motifs upstream from the TATA box are important elements of the SV40 early protomer, *Nucleic Acids Res.* **11**:2447–2464.

Fromm, M., and Berg, P., 1982, Deletion mapping of DNA regions required for SV40 early region promoter function *in vivo*, *J. Mol. Appl. Genet.* **1**:457–481.

Ghosh, P. K., Lebowitz, P., Frisque, F. J., and Gluzman, Y., 1981, Identification of a promoter component involved in positioning the 5′ termini of simian virus 40 early mRNAs, *Proc. Natl. Acad. Sci. U.S.A.* **78**:100–104.

Gidoni, D., Dynan, W. S., and Tjian, R., 1984, Multiple specific contacts between a mammalian transcription factor and its cognate promoters, *Nature (London)* **312**:409–413.

Gidoni, D., Kadonaga, J. T., Barrera-Saldana, H., Takahashi, K., Chambon, P., and Tjian, R., 1985, Bidirectional SV40 transcription mediated by tandem Sp1 binding interactions, *Science* **230**:511–517.

Hansen, U., and Sharp, P. A., 1983, Sequences controlling *in vitro* transcription of SV40 promoters, *Eur. Mol. Biol. Org. J.* **2**:2293–2303.

Jones, K. A., and Tjian, R., 1985, Sp1 binds to promoter sequences and activates HSV "immediate-early" gene transcription *in vitro, Nature (London)* **317**:179–182.

Jones, K. A., Yamamoto, K. R., and Tjian, R., 1985, Two distinct transcription factors bind to the HSV thymidine kinase promoter *in vitro, Cell* **42**:559–572.

Kadonaga, J. T., and Tjian, R., 1986, Affinity purification of sequence-specific DNA binding proteins, *Proc. Natl. Acad. Sci. U.S.A.* **83**:5889–5893.

Kadonaga, J. T., Jones, K. A., and Tjian, R., 1986, Promoter-specific activation of RNA polymerase II transcription by Sp1, *Trends Biochem.* **11**:20–23.

Lebowitz, P., and Ghosh, P. K., 1982, Initiation and regulation of simian virus 40 early transcription *in vitro, J. Virol.* **41**:449–461.

Moreau, P., Hen, R., Wasylyk, B., Everett, R., Gaub, M. P., and Chambon, P., 1981, The SV40 72 base pair repeat has a striking effect on gene expression both in SV40 and other chimeric recombinants, *Nucleic Acids Res.* **9**:6047–6067.

Myers, R. M., Rio, D. C., Robbins, A. K., and Tjian, R., 1981, SV40 gene expression is modulated by the cooperative binding of T antigen to DNA, *Cell* **25**:373–384.

Parker, C. S., and Topol, J., 1984, A *Drosophila* RNA polymerase II transcription factor specific for the heat shock gene binds to the regulatory site of an hsp 70 gene, *Cell* **37**:273–283.

Pelham, H. R. B., 1982, A regulatory upstream promoter element in the *Drosophila* Hsp heat shock gene, *Cell* **30**:517–528.

Picard, D., and Schaffner, W., 1984, A lymphocyte-specific enhancer in the mouse immunoglobulin gene, *Nature (London)* **307**:80–82.

Queen, C., and Baltimore, D., 1983, Immunoglobulin gene transcription is activated by downstream sequence elements, *Cell* **33**:741–748.

Rio, D. C., and Tjian, R., 1984, Multiple control elements involved in the initiation of SV40 late transcription, *J. Mol. Appl. Genet.* **2**:423–435.

Sawadogo, M., and Roeder, R. G., 1985, Interaction of a gene-specific transcription factor with the adenovirus major late promoter upstream of the TATA box region, *Cell* **43**:165–175.

Stuart, G. W., Searle, P. F., Chen, H. Y., Brinster, R. L., and Palmiter, R. D., 1984, A 12-base-pair DNA motif that is repeated several times in metallothionein gene promoters confers metal regulation to a heterologous gene, *Proc. Natl. Acad. Sci. U.S.A.* **81**:7318–7322.

Weil, P. A., Luse, D. S., Segall, J., and Roeder, R. G., 1979, Selective and accurate initiation of transcription at the Ad2 major late promoter in a soluble system dependent on purified RNA polymerase II and DNA, *Cell* **18**:469–484.

8

Chromatin Structure Near an Expressed Gene

GARY FELSENFELD, BEVERLY M. EMERSON,
P. DAVID JACKSON, CATHERINE D. LEWIS,
JOANNE E. HESSE, MICHAEL R. LIEBER,
and JOANNE M. NICKOL

1. Introduction

The DNA within eukaryotic nuclei is complexed with basic proteins called *histones* to form a compact structure. Although little is known about the way in which higher orders of compaction are achieved, the two lowest levels of DNA packing in chromatin are relatively well understood. The fundamental chromatin subunit is the *nucleosome*. The central portion of each nucleosome is the *chromatosome*, which contains 165 base pairs (bp) of DNA wrapped in two superhelical turns about an octamer of histones. Each chromatosome is connected to its neighbor by a segment of linker DNA, the length of which varies from about 10 to 80 bp. The next level of compaction requires that the lineas polynucleosome filament be folded to form a fiber 30 nm in diameter. Most evidence suggests that this is a solenoidal structure in which the filament is supercoiled to give a fiber with about six nucleosomes per turn (Finch and Klug, 1976; Felsenfeld and McGhee, 1986).

Work in our laboratory using electric dichroism has provided information about the orientation of the chromatosomes within this structure.

GARY FELSENFELD, BEVERLY M. EMERSON, P. DAVID JACKSON, CATHERINE D. LEWIS, JOANNE E. HESSE, MICHAEL R. LIEBER, and JOANNE M. NICKOL • Laboratory of Molecular Biology, National Institute of Diabetes, and Digestive and Kidney Diseases, National Institutes of Health, Bethesda, Maryland 20892.

When combined with data from other physical measurements, the dichroism results lead to the conclusion that individual chromatosomes must be arranged radially within the solenoid, with a tilt of about 25° relative to its long axis (Fig. 1).

Given the compact nature of the 30-nm fiber, it is clear that when a eukaryotic gene is expressed, the chromatin structure containing the gene must be disrupted. In this chapter, we consider the ways in which the chromatin of an expressed gene is altered as a precondition or a consequence of its expression.

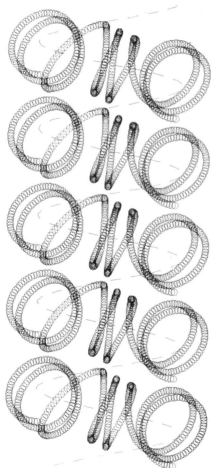

Figure 1. Proposed model for the path of DNA within the 30-nm chromatin fiber of chicken erythrocyte nuclei (McGhee *et al.*, 1983). The chromatosomes (two turns of duplex, more tightly supercoiled) are connected by linker DNA, and the entire polynucleosome filament is wound into a solenoid with six nucleosomes per turn. Only the front nucleosomes of each turn are shown.

2. Results

During the past several years, we have studied the chromatin structure of the adult beta (β^A) globin gene in chicken erythrocytes. It is known from work in a number of laboratories that a considerable fraction of the globin gene copies are packaged in nucleosomes; recent studies of our own (P. D. Jackson and G. Felsenfeld, unpublished data) show that these nucleosomes have physical properties quite similar to those of bulk nucleosomes or of nucleosomes containing transcriptionally inactive genes.

In cells in which the globin gene is expressed, the gene can be distinguished by an unusual sensitivity to nucleases. The sensitivity takes two forms: The first kind, originally described by Weintraub and his collaborators (Weintraub and Groudine, 1976), extends over the entire domain containing the gene and for a considerable distance on either side of it (Fig. 2). Typically, such a domain is about 10-fold more sensitive than inactive chromatin to digestion by deoxyribonuclease (DNase) I. The active globin chromatin also displays a second kind of response of nucleases: In the 5′ flanking region, confined to a domain about 200 bp long, is a DNA segment that is perhaps 100-fold more sensitive to digestion than inactive chromatin (McGhee *et al.*, 1981). The hypersensitive behavior is not found in 5-day-old embryonic red cells, in which the gene is not expressed, but it is found in 9-day-old embryonic red cells. A second hypersensitive domain has been identified in the 3′ flanking region; it is present in 5-day embryonic red cells as well as at later stages (McGhee *et al.*, 1981).

We have focused considerable attention on the 5′ hypersensitive domain. Nuclease probes have allowed us to define its limits: It extends about 200 bp in the 5′ direction, starting approximately at nucleotide −50 relative to the site of transcription initiation. Within this region is a pair of *Msp*I restriction sites, 114 bp apart. When nuclei from 9-day to adult red cells are treated with *Msp*I, the 114-bp fragment is released from the nuclei in greater than 50% yield. Thus, most or all of the gene copies are in a hypersensitive state. Furthermore, the fact that both sites are accessible shows that a normal nucleosome cannot be present, since a nucleosome protects at least 145 bp of DNA from nuclease attack.

We speculated that the absence of a nucleosome might reflect the presence of other proteins binding to the region. To test this possibility, we reconstituted histones onto plasmids containing the globin gene in the pres-

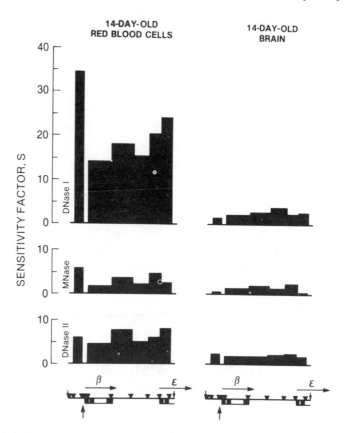

Figure 2. Relative sensitivity to nucleases of chick globin genes in nuclei from 14-day embryonic red cells and brain. The entire β-globin gene, and a portion of the ε-globin gene,
are included (see map at bottom). (↑) Position of the 5′ hypersensitive domain. From
Wood and Felsenfeld (1982).

ence of erythrocyte nuclear extracts. A significant fraction of such complexes show the same preferential accessibility of the *Msp*I sites in the
5′ flanking region seen *in vivo*. These nuclear extracts thus contain factors capable of preventing a nucleosome from binding to the hypersensitive domain.

Our subsequent investigations have been devoted to a search for these
factors. We have made use of filter binding assays (Emerson and Felsenfeld, 1984) and more recently of footprinting techniques (Emerson *et al.*,
1985). In this way (Figs. 3 and 4), we have identified in the 5′ hypersensitive domain two regions that are complexed to proteins other than

histones. The two regions are quite different in sequence: One includes a string of 16 G residues, while the other, located about 15 bp 3′ of the first, contains an inverted repeat in which 18 of 25 bases are potentially paired. At the 3′ end of the inverted repeat is a consensus sequence of 10 nucleotides that has been identified in the promoter regions of adult β-globin genes of many organisms and that has been shown in transient expression assays to have a stimulatory effect on transcription (Dierks *et al.*, 1983; Charnay *et al.*, 1984).

There are at least two and probably three different proteins involved in this binding activity. We have shown that when the two regions described above are separately cloned, their characteristic footprints can be generated independently of one another (Emerson *et al.*, 1985). Quite recently (unpublished data), we have found that under some circumstances, nuclear preparations from embryonic red cells may be preferentially depleted of the palindrome-sequence binding factors. This establishes that the factors binding to the G-string and the palindrome are distinct; furthermore, it seems likely that at least two distinct proteins are associated with the palindrome and the consensus sequence located immediately downstream.

We have compared the results obtained *in vitro* with the pattern of binding within nuclei. To carry out these experiments, we have devised a method of intranuclear footprinting (Jackson and Felsenfeld, 1985) that is an extension of the technique that employs S1 nuclease to identify the 5′ ends of RNA transcripts (Berk and Sharp, 1977). We have found that within adult red-cell nuclei, the palindrome and consensus sequences are clearly protected; we found with somewhat less certainty that the string of G residues also seems to be protected. Thus, factors that are observed to bind *in vitro* are bound within the nucleus as well.

Although we have obtained information about the structure of the 5′ hypersensitive domain, it is obviously important to have a means of assessing biological function as well. We have recently found that it is possible to study globin-gene expression by transfecting DNA sequences into primary embryonic erythrocytes (Hesse *et al.*, 1986). The method uses DEAE–Dextran–DNA complexes to introduce DNA into the cell for transient expression studies, but first the cells are osmotically shocked by exposure to ammonium chloride. This treatment ultimately leads to high and reproducible levels of expression.

When this method is used to introduce a plasmid in which the β^A-globin gene promoter is fused to the *cat* structural gene, low levels of chlo-

Gary Felsenfeld et al.

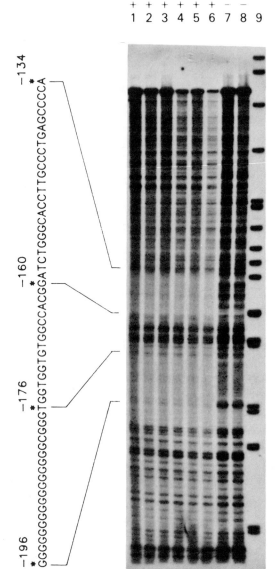

Figure 3. DNase I footprints of partially purified factors from adult chicken red-cell nuclei on DNA of the βA-globin 5′ flanking region. Two distinct protected domains can be seen. From Emerson *et al.* (1985).

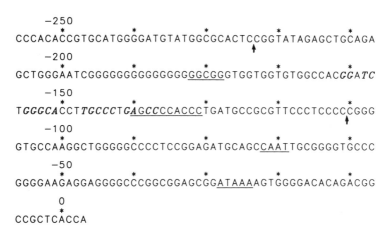

Figure 4. Sequence of the chicken β^A-globin gene 5' flanking region. The complementary bases of the inverted repeat are shown in italics; the consensus sequence common to adult β-globin promoters is contiguous with the inverted repeat and is underlined. The 3' end of the string of G residues, the CAAT sequence, and the TATA sequence are also underlined. (↑) *Msp*I sites that can be cut to release this segment of DNA from the nucleus. From Emerson *et al.* (1985).

ramphenicol acetyltransferase (CAT) expression are observed (Hesse *et al.*, 1986). To determine whether downstream elements of the globin gene might be important for transcription, we examined the effect of introducing the coding region of the gene, as well as sequences in the gene's 3' flanking region. These were added 3' of the *cat* gene and simian virus 40 (SV40) splicing and termination signals (see Fig. 5). Relative to the construction containing the promoter region only, a 6-fold stimulation of CAT activity was seen in transfected 9-day embryonic cells when both the coding region and the 3' flanking region were added. Analysis of additional constructions showed that the stimulatory effect is contained only in the 3' flanking region and resides entirely within a 479-bp sequence that begins 110 bp 3' of the globin gene's polyadenylation signal (Fig. 5, segment E).

Schaffner had previously reported that the 3' flanking region of the chicken β^A-globin gene contains an enhancer element [personal communication (quoted in Hesse *et al.*, 1986)]. Our work confirms this observation. When segment E is fused directly to the *cat*/SV40 sequence preceded by the globin promoter, an 80-fold stimulation of CAT expres-

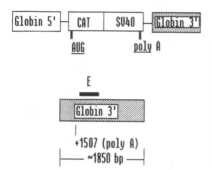

Figure 5. Schematic diagram of plasmids in which the 5′ promoter of the chick β^A-globin gene is fused to the gene for CAT and the SV40 splice and polyadenylation sites. Various portions of the globin gene are then introduced at the 3′ end. Segment E, which begins 110 bp 3′ of the β^A-globin polyadenylation signal, has the properties of an enhancer. From Hesse *et al.* (1986).

sion is observed. As expected for an enhancer, the activity is observed when the E segment is inserted in either orientation or when it is moved to a position directly upstream of the promoter (Hesse *et al.*, 1986).

As noted above, there is a second hypersensitive domain downstream of the globin gene. Within our present limits of resolution, this domain appears to be located in the region that contains the enhancer activity. It seems likely that as in the case of the 5′ domain, specific protein factors will be bound within this region.

3. Discussion

Our experiments show that factors present in erythrocyte nuclear extracts can prevent the binding of histones to the 5′ flanking region of the β^A-globin gene. We have partially purified from the extract specific factors that bind to the DNA of this region. It is reasonable to speculate that some or all of these factors may be involved in the generation of the hypersensitive domain *in vivo*, although it must be kept in mind that these are impure preparations, and therefore the assays for binding and that for exclusion of histones may reflect the action of different components.

The simple model for the generation of a hypersensitive domain suggested by these experiments was originally proposed by Brown and his co-workers (Bogenhagen *et al.*, 1982) to explain the action of the *Xenopus 5S* gene transcription factor, TFIIIA. In the case of TFIIIA, addition of the factor prior to addition of histones resulted in stimulation of transcription, while complexes formed by adding histones before TFIIIA were inactive. Brown suggested that activation *in vivo* requires the binding of the factor to its site on the *5S* gene at a point in replication prior to the laying down of new histones on DNA. We might suppose similarly that the exclusion of histones from the globin 5′ flanking region occurs *in vivo* during replication and that the binding of the factors we have identified (or others like them) is responsible.

This is not the only possible mechanism for generation of a hypersensitive domain. Weintraub has proposed that the DNA sequence within a hypersensitive domain may be capable of assuming an unusual secondary structure (Larsen and Weintraub, 1982; Weintraub, 1983). This possibility is suggested by the presence in many such domains of sequences that, when inserted in supercoiled plasmids, are sensitive to digestion by the single-strand-specific S1 nuclease. Such structures might prevent the binding of normal nucleosomes, and one might well imagine that the extent to which the structures form within the nucleus is modulated by the amount of local supercoiling.

The string of 16 G residues in the 5′ flanking region of the β^A-globin gene is sensitive to S1 nuclease when it is present in supercoiled plasmids (Nickol and Felsenfeld, 1983). The nature of the structure that gives rise to this sensitivity is the subject of considerable debate (Nickol and Felsenfeld, 1983; Cantor and Efstradiatis, 1984; Pulleyblank *et al.*, 1985; Lyamichev *et al.*, 1986). It is possible that different structures are preferentially stabilized in response to varying salt concentration and pH. Since no comparable high-resolution analysis has been made of the pattern of S1 sensitivity of DNA within the nucleus, it is not known whether the sites of intranuclear S1 cuts occur within the same sequence.

On the basis of our own intranuclear footprinting studies of adult red-cell nuclei, it seems likely that the entire sequence of G residues is covered by nonhistone protein. In contrast, the oligo (G) sequence may be exposed in oviduct nuclei (unpublished data), in which the gene is not expressed, although most of the hypersensitive domain is covered by protein (perhaps a nucleosome). It is possible that the unknown structure that gives rise to S1 sensitivity also serves to reduce the affinity of histone octamers in its neighborhood and that this reduced affinity makes it easier for the specific binding proteins to win the competition with histones. It should be noted that long homopolymer duplexes can exclude nucleosomes even in the absence of supercoiling (Kunkel and Martinson, 1981).

In cells in which it is expressed, the β^A-globin gene is bounded at either end by domains in which the regular chromatin structure is perturbed. Between, and probably beyond, these domains, a considerable number of nucleosomes are bound. At salt concentrations of 50 mM, these are sufficient to partially refold the polynucleosome filament, but there is evidence that the filament may not be able to fold into a fully compact 30-nm fiber (Kimura *et al.*, 1983; Fisher and Felsenfeld, 1986). This lack of compaction may be responsible for the general nuclease sensitivity that extends over the gene and its surroundings. Although we cannot yet be certain of the order of events within the cell, it is possible that the generation of hypersensitive domains is an early step in the formation of active chromatin and that these domains then serve as the nucleation points for the unfolding of the fiber.

References

Berk, A. J., and Sharp, P. A., 1977, Sizing and mapping of early adenovirus mRNAs by gel electrophoresis of S1 endonuclease digested hybrids, *Cell* **12**:721–732.

Bogenhagen, D. F., Wormington, W. M., and Brown, D. D. 1982, Stable transcription complexes of Xenopus 5S RNA genes: A means to maintain the differentiated state, *Cell* **28**:413–421.

Cantor, C. R., and Efstradiatis, A., 1984, Possible structure of homopurine homopyrimidine S1 hypersensitive sites, *Nucleic Acids Res.* **12**:8059–8072.

Charnay, P., Treisman, R., Mellon, P., Chao, M., Axel, R., and Maniatis, T., 1984, Differences in human α- and β-globin gene expression in mouse erythroleukemia cells: The role of intragenic sequences, *Cell* **38**:251–263.

Dierks, P., van Ooyen, A., Cochran, M. D., Dobkin, C., Reiser, J., and Weissman, C., 1983, Three regions upstream from the Cap site are required for efficient and accurate transcription of the rabbit beta-globin gene in mouse 3T6 cells, *Cell* **32**:695–706.

Emerson, B. M., and Felsenfeld, G., 1984, Specific factor conferring nuclease hypersensitivity at the 5′ end of the chicken adult β-globin gene, *Proc. Natl. Acad. Sci. U.S.A.* **81**:95–99.

Emerson, B. M., Lewis, C. D., and Felsenfeld, G., 1985, Interaction of specific nuclear factors with the nuclease-hypersensitive region of the chicken adult β-globin gene: Nature of the binding domain, *Cell* **41**:21–30.

Felsenfeld, G., and McGhee, J. D., 1986, Structure of the 30 nm chromatin fiber, *Cell* **44**:375–377.

Finch, J. T., and Klug, A., 1976, Solenoidal model for superstructure in chromatin, *Proc. Natl. Acad. Sci. U.S.A.* **73**:1897–1901.

Fisher, E. A. and Felsenfeld, G. 1986, A comparison of the folding of β-globin and ovalbumin gene-containing chromatin from chicken oviduct and erythrocytes, *Biochemistry* (in press).

Hesse, J. E., Nickol, J. M., Lieber, M. R., and Felsenfeld, G., 1986, Regulated gene expression in transfected primary chicken erythrocytes, *Proc. Natl. Acad. Sci. U.S.A.* **83**:4312–4316.

Jackson, P. D., and Felsenfeld, G., 1985, A method for mapping intranuclear protein–

DNA interactions and its application to a nuclease hypersensitive site, *Proc. Natl. Acad. Sci. U.S.A.* **82**:2296–2300.

Kimura, T., Mills, F. C., Allan, J., and Gould, H., 1983, Selective unfolding of erythroid chromatin in the region of the active beta-globin gene, *Nature (London)* **306**:709–712.

Kunkel, G. R., and Martinson, H. G., 1981, Nucleosomes will not form on double-stranded RNA or over poly(dA)•poly(dT) tracts in recombinant DNA, *Nucleic Acids Res.* **9**:6869–6888.

Larsen, A., and Weintraub, H., 1982, An altered DNA conformation detected by S1 nuclease occurs at specific regions in active chick globin chromatin, *Cell* **29**:609–622.

Lyamichev, V. I., Mirkin, S. M., and Frank-Kamenetskii, M.D., 1986, Structures of homopurine-homopyrimidine tract in superhelical DNA, *J. Biomol. Struct. Dynam.* **3**:667–669.

McGhee, J. D., Wood, W. I., Dolan, M., Engel, J. D., and Felsenfeld, G., 1981, A 200 base pair region at the 5′ end of the chicken adult β-globin gene is accessible to nuclease digestion, *Cell* **27**:45–55.

McGhee, J. D., Nickol, J. M., Felsenfeld, G., and Rau, D. C., 1983, Higher order structure of chromatin: Orientation of nucleosomes within the 30 nm chromatin solenoid is independent of species and spacer length, *Cell* **33**:831–841.

Nickol, J. M., and Felsenfeld, G., 1983, DNA conformation at the 5′ end of the chicken adult β-globin gene, *Cell* **35**:467–477.

Pulleyblank, D. E., Haniford, D. B., and Morgan, A. R., 1985, A structural basis for S1 nuclease sensitivity of double-stranded DNA, *Cell* **42**:271–280.

Weintraub, H., 1983, A dominant role for DNA secondary structure in forming hypersensitive structures in chromatin, *Cell* **32**:1191–1203.

Weintraub, H., and Groudine, M., 1976, Chromosomal subunits in active genes have an altered conformation, *Science* **193**:848–856.

Wood, W. I., and Felsenfeld, G., 1982, Chromatin structure of the chicken β-globin region: Sensitivity to DNase I, micrococcal nuclease, and DNase II, *J. Biol. Chem.* **257**:7730–7736.

9

Specificity of Gene Expression and Insertional Mutagenesis in Transgenic Mice

HEINER WESTPHAL, JASPAL S. KHILLAN,
KATHLEEN A. MAHON, PAUL A. OVERBEEK,
ANA B. CHEPELINSKY, JORAM PIATIGORSKY,
AZRIEL SCHMIDT, and BENOIT DE CROMBRUGGHE

1. Introduction

Transgenic mice constitute an ideal system for determining the spatial and temporal control of gene expression in every conceivable tissue of the mammalian organism. A wide variety of gene constructs have been inserted in the mouse germ line, and the initial data compiled with this system have recently been reviewed by Gordon and Ruddle (1985) and by Palmiter and Brinster (1985). One of the most important conclusions from this initial work has been that expression of transferred genes may be directed to specific organs and tissues of the transgenic mouse, irrespective of the site of integration in the genome. In addition, a number of chimeric genes containing a 5′ flanking region of gene A and the coding sequence of gene B were found to express gene product B in the target tissue

HEINER WESTPHAL, JASPAL S. KHILLAN, KATHLEEN A. MAHON, and PAUL A.
OVERBEEK • Laboratory of Molecular Genetics, National Institute of Child Health and Human Development, National Institutes of Health, Bethesda, Maryland 20892. *ANA B. CHEPELINSKY and JORAM PIATIGORSKY* • Laboratory of Molecular and Developmental Biology, National Eye Institute, National Institutes of Health, Bethesda, Maryland 20892. *AZRIEL SCHMIDT and BENOIT DE CROMBRUGGHE* • Laboratory of Molecular Biology, Division of Cancer Biology and Diagnosis, National Cancer Institute, National Institutes of Health, Bethesda, Maryland 20892.

determined by gene A. Examples from our own laboratories that cor-
roborate this fact include chimeric gene constructs composed of untranslated control regions of the mouse αA crystallin gene, mouse α2(I) collagen gene, or avian Rous sarcoma virus (RSV) and the bacterial sequence
that encodes chloramphenicol acetyltransferase (CAT). In each instance,
the upstream sequences exerted specific spatial and temporal controls on
CAT expression in the transgenic mouse. A case in point is the αA crystallin control region that was found to produce the CAT enzyme selectively in the lens of the eye (Overbeek *et al.*, 1985).

We needed this type of specificity to address a problem of medical
relevance, posed by the apparent tumor immunity of the eye lens. Lens
tumors are virtually unknown in nature (for a review, see Piatigorsky,
1981). We wondered, however, whether it would be possible to induce
such tumors by inserting in the mouse a chimeric gene consisting of the
αA crystallin control region fused to a sequence that encodes a known
tumor antigen. The construct we made contains the coding region for the
simian virus 40 (SV40) tumor antigens shown to be tumorigenic in transgenic mice (Brinster *et al.*, 1984; Hanahan, 1985; Palmiter *et al.*, 1985).
We will describe herein how mice carrying and expressing SV40 large
tumor (large-T) antigen under the control of the αA of crystallin 5' flanking region do indeed develop lens tumors and a specific disease pattern.

Irrespective of the functions they encode, foreign genes inserted into
the mouse germ line may also act as insertional mutagens (for a review,
see Marx, 1985). We will present one such case from our collection of
transgenic strains, in which insertion of the foreign gene caused a recessive mutation that manifests itself as a special type of limb deformity.

2. Experiments and Results

Three different experiments with transgenic mice are described herein.
In the first experiment, we measured controls exerted on the bacterial CAT
gene by various 5' flanking sequences. The developmental timing and the
tissue specificity of expression of two such chimeric constructs, αA
crystallin–CAT and α2(I) collagen–CAT, reflected closely the temporal
and spatial regulation of the genuine mouse genes from which the 5' flanks
were derived. A third construct, RSV–CAT, containing long terminal repeat (LTR) sequences of an avian sarcoma virus, was found to be expressed predominantly in organs rich in muscle, bone, and connective tis-

sue. There are parallels between this tissue specificity and the disease specificity of the intact RSV.

The second experiment demonstrates that the eye lens, which is naturally refractory to tumor formation, can undergo malignant transformation in a transgenic mouse. Several mice carrying a chimeric αA crystallin–SV40 large-T antigen construct were obtained. Each of these developed a vascularized tumor in both lenses. Both the lens tissue and cells cultured *in vitro* from this tissue were found to produce SV40 large-T antigen and the lens crystallins. Animals carrying the tumor are able to pass this trait on to progeny. Maintenance of the trait has been difficult because the animals die at a young age. Metastasis has so far been detected in only one animal.

A case of apparent insertional mutagenesis is the subject of the third experiment. We noticed a recessive trait of syndactyly (a fusion of phalanges in all four feet) in a strain carrying the RSV–CAT construct. The trait cosegregates with the gene insert and appears to be allelic to a previously described spontaneously occurring syndactyly that has been mapped in chromosome 18.

2.1. Spatial and Temporal Control of Marker Gene Expression in Mice Carrying αA Crystallin–Chloramphenicol Acetyltransferase, α2(I) Collagen–Chloramphenicol Acetyltransferase, or Rous Sarcoma Virus–Chloramphenicol Acetyltransferase Chimeric Genes

In the experiments described below, fusion genes were introduced into the mouse germ line by zygote microinjection (Gordon and Ruddle, 1985; Palmiter and Brinster, 1985). The resulting transgenic strains were assayed for CAT expression in various tissues and at different times of pre- and postnatal development. The bacterial CAT gene product served as an easy-to-score marker for gene expression directed by individual upstream sequences. We have published detailed accounts of our experiments with the αA crystallin–CAT gene (Overbeek *et al.*, 1985), the α2(I) collagen–CAT gene (Khillan *et al.*, 1986), and the RSV–CAT gene (Overbeek *et al.*, 1986) and will confine ourselves here to summarizing our conclusions.

Figure 1 provides a synopsis of the tissue specificity exerted by the three upstream sequences. As can be seen in this organ screen of three representative transgenic animals, the αA crystallin gene sequence directs CAT expression selectively to the eye. Main target organs for the other two constructs are the tail [a2(I) collagen–CAT] and muscle and bone (RSV–CAT). The upstream sequences must play a decisive role in this tissue selectivity because the downstream sequences, consisting of the bacterial CAT gene and of SV40 splicing and polyadenylation signals, are the same in each case.

Specifically, 409 base pairs of the mouse αA crystallin 5' flanking sequences (-364 to $+45$) were sufficient to direct CAT expression selectively to the lens fibers and epithelia of the transgenic animal. An extensive screen of over 20 organs and tissues failed to detect any other site of CAT expression. CAT activity was first detected in embryonic eyes at day 12.5 of gestation. Both the timing and the tissue specificity of CAT expression coincided well with that of the endogenous αA crystallin gene. Likewise, a 5' flanking region, -2000 to $+54$, of the α2(I) collagen gene of the mouse directed CAT gene expression predominantly to the tail, an organ rich in connective tissue. CAT expression was detected as early as day 8 of embryonic development. Again, both the target and the timing of expression of the chimeric collagen–CAT gene in our transgenic animals reflected that of the endogenous α2(I) collagen gene.

With the third construct, RSV–CAT, the task was not to establish parallels of regulation between the chimeric gene and an endogenous one. Rather, our aim was to determine the spatial and temporal regulation of control sequences derived from a virus that is actually foreign to the mammalian organism. RSV is an avian virus, albeit one that can also induce sarcomas in rodents.

The sequences fused to CAT were derived from the terminal part of the viral genome and were known to contain transcriptional promoter and enhancer elements. We obtained five mouse strains carrying and expressing RSV–CAT. The spectrum of tissue specificity of CAT expression in each of these independent strains is quite similar to the one shown in Fig. 1, with the main targets of expression being organs rich in muscle, bone, and connective tissue. These same tissues are also, of course, targets of oncogenesis in birds and rodents infected with the intact RSV virus particle. It is therefore tempting to envisage a connection between the target-tissue specificity of RSV control sequences and the viral disease specificity. Elevated levels of viral gene expression, including *src*, in tissues of mesenchymal provenance may be the molecular origin of the sarcomas caused by RSV. Concerning the timing of expression, it was interesting to note that CAT activity peaked well after birth, indicating that the RSV control sequences contained in our RSV–CAT construct are effectively shut off at earlier stages of development.

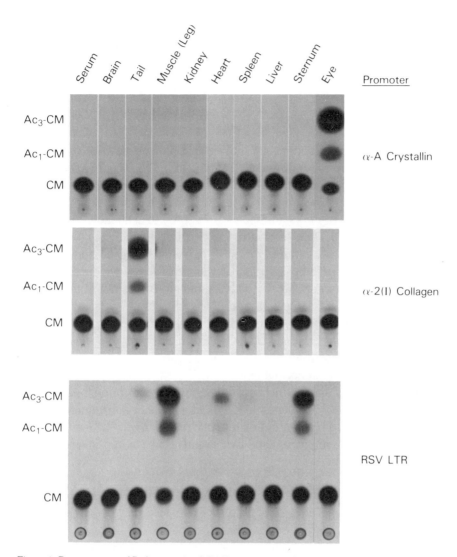

Figure 1. Promoter-specified patterns of CAT gene expression in transgenic mice. Organ screens for CAT activity were performed on three individual F_1 animals expressing, respectively, the αA crystallin–CAT, the α2(I) collagen–CAT, or the RSV–CAT insert. Acetylated forms of chloramphenicol (Ac_1-CM, Ac_3-CM) indicate the presence of acetyltransferase in the respective tissues. For details of the assay, see Overbeek *et al.* (1985).

In conclusion, the results obtained with our three chimeric gene constructs have validated our approach of using the CAT marker to screen for specific signals of gene control. Knowledge gained from this type of screening procedure is a prerequisite for the type of experimental question addressed below.

2.2. Dominant Lens Tumors Caused by an αA Crystallin–Simian Virus 40 Large-T Antigen Fusion Gene

In the previous section, we showed that defined upstream sequences of the mouse αA crystallin gene, linked to the CAT coding sequences, direct marker expression to the lens and that expression begins at an early fetal stage. Herein, we discuss a construct in which the same upstream sequences of the αA crystallin gene were fused to sequences that encode SV40 early genes. The expectation was that large-T antigen would be expressed in the lens of transgenic mice carrying this gene construct and that expression would begin at an early stage of lens development. However, since lens tumors are virtually unknown, it was not at all predictable whether large T-antigen expression could result in malignant proliferation of lens tissue in these transgenic mice.

Our initial observations of seven F_o animals carrying one or more copies of the chimeric gene were quite uniform. Each of these animals displayed strikingly abnormal lenses, these being apparent as soon as the newborn animals opened their eyes. Eventually, lens tumors developed. The animals died young, at about 3 months of age, a circumstance that made the genetic preservation of this phenotype difficult. We were successful, however, in propagating two strains. Some of the salient features

--→

Figure 2. Lens tumor in mice carrying the αA crystallin–SV40 large-T antigen chimeric gene. (A) Lenses of a normal animal *(right)* and a mouse bearing the αA crystallin–SV40 large-T antigen construct. *(left)* The lens of the transgenic animal is opaque and yellow. (B) Cross section of the lens tumor of a $3^1/2$-month-old F_0 animal. The lens mass is composed of many small, mitotically active cells (see arrow) and a few abnormal, terminally differentiated "balloon cells" (b) and is infiltrated by blood vessels (v). The lens cells in the bottom right corner have grown out of the capsule (c) that normally encompasses the lens. Giemsa stain. Scale bar: 50 μm. (C) Immunofluorescent staining of lens tumor tissue with a monoclonal antibody against SV40 large-T antigen, showing the typical nuclear location of large-T antigen. Scale bar: 50 μm.

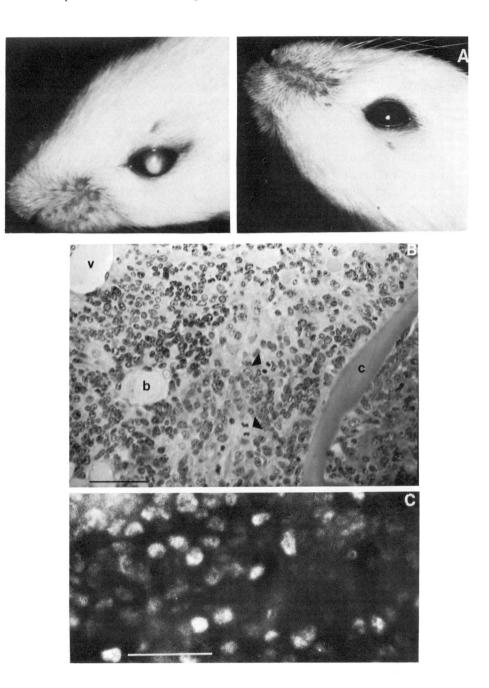

of the lens tumor are described below. Details of this work will be published elsewhere (K. H. Mahon, A. B. Chepelinsky, J. S. Khillan, P. A. Overbeek, J. Piatgorsky, and H. Westphal, manuscript submitted).

The lens tumor is easily discernible in Fig. 2A. In a 3-month-old animal, we found that the tumor was well vascularized and that it had grown out of the lens capsule. A cross section (Fig. 2B) revealed lens cells of aberrant morphology. Nuclear SV40 large-T antigen was readily detected by immunofluorescent staining both in lens tissue (Fig. 2C) and in a cell line derived therefrom. Some but not all of the lens cells continued to synthesize lens crystallins. A thorough postmortem examination of mice carrying the lens tumor revealed malignancies elsewhere in the body. For example, in one animal we detected a pea-sized tumor behind the right eye. A cell line derived from this metastasis was also found to contain SV40 large-T antigen.

We conclude that the 5′ flanking αA crystallin sequence directs SV40 large-T-antigen production specifically in the lens and that the expression is early, possibly coinciding with that of the genuine αA crystallin gene. The events between induction of SV40 large-T antigen and the development of a lens tumor and an ultimately fatal disease are topics of our present studies.

2.3. Syndactyly in a Rous Sarcoma Virus–Chloramphenicol Acetyltransferase Strain

Syndactyly, a phenotype of fused digits, was detected in one of our transgenic strains carrying the RSV–CAT chimeric gene insert. About one fourth of the offspring resulting from $F_1 \times F_1$ crosses were affected, suggesting that manifestation of the phenotype requires homozygosity at the site of insertion. Figure 3 displays this limb deformity, which comprises fusion of phalanges between the second and third or third and fourth digits in the fore and hind feet. Affected animals are viable and fertile. Extensive breeding of the strain confirmed cosegregation of the syndactyly and the RSV–CAT marker.

One of the spontaneously arising cases of syndactyly in the mouse, termed sy^{fp}, is related to ours with respect to both inheritance pattern and phenotype (Hummel and Chapman, 1971). The sy^{fp} mutation has been mapped to chromosome 18. We crossed homozygous sy^{fp} animals with our strain and obtained offspring with syndactyly that was indistinguishable from that of either parent. This result is expected if both mutations belong to the same complementation group and strongly suggests that the genetic defect in our strain is allelic to that of sy^{fp}.

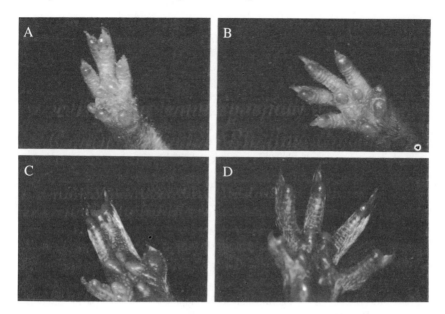

Figure 3. Syndactyly in a transgenic mouse carrying the RSV–CAT construct. (A) Front foot and (C) hind foot of an F_2 mouse showing the fused-toe phenotype. (B) Front foot and (D) hind foot of an apparently normal sibling. Reprinted from Overbeek *et al.* (1986) with the permission of *Science*; copyright 1986 by the AAAS.

Remarkably, another case of limb deformity has been reported in a strain of transgenic mice (Woychik *et al.*, 1985). The mutation is also recessive and involves more extensive bone fusions in all four extremities. It appears to be allelic with *ld*, a spontaneously occurring limb deformity, mapped to chromosome 2.

The gene inserts in both strains can be used as molecular markers for the purpose of cloning and characterizing the affected genes. This constitutes an important first step toward a molecular understanding of the control of limb formation in the mouse.

References

Brinster, R. L., Chen, H. Y., Messing, A., van Dyke, T., Levine, A. J., and Palmiter, R. D., 1984, Transgenic mice harboring SV40 T-antigen genes develop characteristic brain tumors, *Cell* **37:**367–379.

Gordon, J. W., and Ruddle, F. H., 1985, DNA-mediated genetic transformation of mouse embryos and bone marrow—a review, *Gene* **33**:121–136.

Hanahan, D., 1985, Heritable formation of pancreatic β-cell tumours in transgenic mice expressing recombinant insulin/simian virus 40 oncogenes, *Nature* (*London*) **315**:115–122.

Hummel, K. P., and Chapman, D. B., 1971, New mutants, *Mouse News Lett.* **45**:28.

Khillan, J. S., Schmidt, A., Overbeek, P. A., de Crombrugghe, B., and Westphal, H., 1986, Developmental and tissue-specific expression directed by the $\alpha 2$ type I collagen promoter in transgenic mice, *Proc. Natl. Acad. Sci. U.S.A.* **83**:725–729.

Marx, J. L., 1985, Making mutant mice mice by gene transfer, *Science* **228**:1516–1517.

Overbeek, P. A., Chepelinsky, A. B., Khillan, J. S., Piatigorsky, J., and Westphal, H., 1985, Lens-specific expression and developmental regulation of the bacterial chloramphenicol acetyltransferase gene driven by the murine αA-crystallin promoter in transgenic mice, *Proc. Natl. Acad. Sci, U.S.A.* **82**:7815–7819.

Overbeek, P. A., Lai, S.-P., Van Quill, K. R., and Westphal, H., 1986, Tissue specific expression in transgenic mice of a fused gene containing RSV terminal sequences, *Science* **231**:1574–1577.

Palmiter, R. D., and Brinster, R. L., 1985, Transgenic mice, *Cell* **41**:343–345.

Palmiter, R. D., Chen, H. Y., Messing, A., and Brinster, R. L., 1985, SV40 enhancer and large-T antigen are instrumental in development of choroid plexus tumours in transgenic mice, *Nature* (*London*) **316**:457–460.

Piatigorsky, J., 1981, Lens differentiation in vertebrates: A review of cellular and molecular features, *Differentiation* **19**:134–153.

Woychik, R. P., Stewart, T. A., David, L. G., D'Eustachio, P., and Leder, P., 1985, An inherited limb deformity created by insertional mutagenesis in a transgenic mouse, *Nature* (*London*) **318**:36–40.

10

Retroviruses as Insertional Mutagens

RUDOLF JAENISCH and PHILIPPE SORIANO

1. Introduction

Insertional mutagenesis is a powerful tool for isolating and characterizing genes involved in development because it allows the simultaneous mutating and tagging of a gene. In mammals, two approaches have been successful in inducing insertional mutants: Transgenic animals have been generated by inserting either retroviruses or recombinant DNA into the germ line. Experiments with the first approach exposed mouse embryos to retroviruses at different stages of development (Jaenisch, 1976; Jähner and Jaenisch, 1980; Jaenisch *et al.*, 1981), while experiments with the second approach microinjected mouse zygotes with recombinant DNA (Wagner *et al.*, 1983; Palmiter *et al.*, 1984; Woychik *et al.*, 1985; Mark *et al.*, 1985).

This chapter reviews the current status of retrovirus-induced insertional mutagenesis in mice. It summarizes our understanding of the molecular mechanisms involved in virus-induced mutagenesis, based on extensive analysis of a virus insertion into the $\alpha 1$ (I) collagen gene (Jaenisch *et al.*, 1983; Schnieke *et al.*, 1983). These studies are then compared with the known insertional mutations in mice induced by pronuclear injection of DNA.

2. Insertion of Moloney Murine Leukemia Viruses into the Germ Line of Mice

Mouse strains (called Mov substrains) carrying a single Moloney murine leukemia proviral copy (Mo-MuLV) as a Mendelian determinant were

RUDOLF JAENISCH and PHILIPPE SORIANO • Whitehead Institute for Biomedical Research, Massachusetts Institute of Technology, Cambridge, Massachusetts 02142.

derived by exposing mouse embryos to infectious virus at different developmental stages (Table I). To date, approximately 55 transgenic mouse strains have been derived from virus-infected preimplantation embryos (Jaenisch *et al.*, 1981; Soriano and Jaenisch, 1986), whereas four strains have been derived from embryos micro-injected with infectious virus at midgestation (Jaenisch, 1980; Jaenisch *et al.*, 1981; P. Soriano, unpublished data). Although the frequency of germ-line integrations is high in animals derived from infected preimplantation embryos, infection of primordial germ cells with virus at midgestation is a rare event, and so far only four strains, Mov-13 and Mov-43 to -45, have been obtained by this infection protocol.

3. Expression of the Proviral Genome in Mov Substrains of Mice

Our initial efforts attempted to analyze retrovirus–host genome interactions during the course of mammalian development (reviewed in Jaenisch and Jähner, 1984). Our findings can be summarized as follows:

1. A wild-type proviral genome inserted into the genome of the preimplantation embryo or into embryonal carcinoma cells will not be expressed. In contrast, virus microinjected into the embryo after implantation will replicate in cells of all tissues and will efficiently spread throughout the embryo (Jähner *et al.*, 1982).

2. Once the block to virus expression is established at the preimplantation stage, it is maintained throughout later stages of development, even at stages when the somatic cells have become able to support viral replication. This suggests that once transcriptional inactivity is established

Table I. Insertional Mutations Induced by Experimental Infection with Retroviruses[a]

Stage of exposure to virus	Number of strains		Recessive mutations induced		
	Established[b]	Homozygous[c]	Mov strain	Stage of lethality	Affected gene
Preimplantation	55	41	Mov-34	Soon after implantation	?
Postimplantation	4	1	Mov-13	Day 13 of gestation	$\alpha_1(I)$ collagen

[a]This table is a summary of published and unpublished results.
[b]Transgenic mice established as heterozygous lines.
[c]Number of strains that have so far been obtained as homozygous lines.

at an early developmental stage, it is maintained by a *cis*-acting mechanism. The development of viremia, which is seen in a number of strains (Jaenisch *et al.*, 1981), is due to a rare event of virus activation in a small and as yet unidentified population of cells.

3. DNA methylation is likely to be involved in the maintenance, if not in the establishment, of gene inactivity (Stuhlmann *et al.*, 1981; Harbers *et al.*, 1981; Jähner and Jaenisch, 1985a). Retroviruses become *de novo* methylated when introduced into preimplantation mouse embryos, but not when introduced into postimplantation mouse embryos (Jähner *et al.*, 1982). *De novo* methylase activity as defined by these experiments is characteristic of early embryonic cells and is not detected in cells at later developmental stages (Stewart *et al.*, 1982; Gautsch and Wilson, 1983). The activation of silent retroviral genomes by injection of 5-azacytidine into postnatal animals is consistent with the idea that DNA methylation plays an important role in the maintenance of the transcriptional block (Jaenisch *et al.*, 1985a). *De novo* methylation not only may be involved in inactivation of virus expression, but also may be important for virus-induced repression of adjacent host genes, as summarized in the next section.

4. Induction of Two Insertional Mutations

To screen for recessive mutations induced by virus insertion, we have intercrossed mice heterozygous for 43 different Mo-MuLV proviruses and identified homozygous offspring by Southern-blot DNA analysis. We failed to obtain homozygous animals for two integrations, designated as Mov-13 and Mov-34 (see Table I).

Our first mutant mouse strain, designated as Mov-13, was obtained by microinjection of Mo-MuLV into postimplantation mouse embryos (Jaenisch *et al.*, 1983). The virus insertion in this strain caused an embryonic recessive lethal mutation, with death of homozygous embryos at day 13 of gestation. The mutated gene was cloned and identified as coding for the α1 chain of collagen I (Schnieke *et al.*, 1983). This mouse strain was used to analyze the role of collagen in embryonic development (Löhler *et al.*, 1984) and the molecular mechanisms involved in retrovirus-induced insertional mutagenesis. These experiments (reviewed in Jaenisch *et al.*, 1985b) can be sumarized as follows: The virus in the Mov-13 mouse strain has inserted into the first intron of the collagen gene (Harbers *et al.*, 1984), resulting in a complete block of the developmentally regulated activation of collagen transcription. *In vitro* "runoff" transcription studies with isolated nuclei have shown that initiation of transcription is inhibited by the viral insertion (Hartung *et al.*, 1986). Further molecular analyses demonstrated two virus-induced alterations of the mutated gene: (1) the prevention of the appearance of a deoxyribonuclease (DNase)-I-hypersensitive and transcription-associated site during development (Breindl *et al.*, 1984) and (2) *de novo* methylation of collagen sequences flanking the proviral insertion (Jähner and Jaenisch, 1985b). Both these changes are associated with gene inactivity rather than gene transcription. Alterations similar to those observed with Mov-13 mice have been induced by retroviruses carried in the germ line of other mouse strains. It is therefore possible that alterations of chromatin configuration and DNA methylation patterns are causally related to retrovirus-induced mutations.

We have recently identified a second virus-induced recessive lethal mutation. In contrast to Mov-13, the Mov-34 strain was derived from an embryo exposed to virus at the preimplantation stage (Table I). Embryos homozygous at this locus die early after implantation. The cellular sequences flanking the provirus have been cloned with the help of the bacterial *sup F* gene, which is transduced by the virus (Reik *et al.*, 1985). Our first analyses of the mutant locus indicate that no rearrangements of host sequences flanking the provirus have occurred, which is similar to our findings with the Mov-13 mutant.

5. Insertional Mutagenesis by Retroviruses and DNA Injection

Table II summarizes currently known mutations in mice caused by insertional mutagenesis. The table includes some retrovirus-induced mutations obtained in tissue-culture cells for comparison. The published information allows the conclusion that DNA microinjected into the zygote pronucleus is highly mutagenic and that mutations can realistically be estimated to occur in 10–20% of all transgenic mouse strains generated. Mutations caused by DNA injection include three early embryonic lethals (Covarrubias *et al.*, 1985; Mark *et al.*, 1985), a mutation that causes male transmission distortion (Palmiter *et al.*, 1984), and limb deformity (Woychik *et al.*, 1985). In contrast, only one of the 41 Mov mouse strains derived from virus-exposed preimplantation embryos showed evidence of a mutant phenotype (Mov-34). The Mov-13 mouse strain, the other mutant

Table II. Insertional Mutagenesis in Mice

Insertional mutagen	Developmental stage of exposure	Frequency of mutation induced	Affected gene	Insertion of provirus	Mutant phenotype
Retrovirus	Preimplantation embryo	1/41	?	?	Embryonic lethal
	Midgestation embryo	1/2	α1(I) collagen	First intron	Embryonic lethal
	Spontaneous	?	?	Noncoding	Coat color (d)
	Tissue-culture cells	Low	src	First intron	Reversion of transformation
		?	p-53	First intron	Tumor rejection
		?	κ-Light chain	First intron	Decreased IgG synthesis
		Low	β-Microglobulin	First exon or intron	No protein expression
		Low	*hprt*	Intron	HPRT-
DNA	Zygote pronucleus (microinjection)	10–20%	?		Embryonic lethals
		?			Transmission distortion
		?			Limb deformity

obtained by experimental retrovirus injection, was derived from a primordial germ cell infected at the midgestation stage. The mode of infection by which the spontaneous mutation at the dilute locus (Jenkins *et al.*, 1981) was generated is not known.

Information on the possible mechanism(s) involved in insertional mutagenesis is available so far only for retrovirus-induced mutations. In the most extensively studied mutant, the Mov-13 mouse strain, the virus has inserted into noncoding sequences in the first intron of the collagen gene, which results in a block of gene transcription. Molecular analyses demonstrate two virus-induced alterations of the mutated gene: (1) the prevention of the appearance of a DNase-I-hypersensitive and transcription-associated site during embryonic development and (2) *de novo* methylation of sequences flanking the proviral insertion. Both these changes are associated with gene inactivity, rather than with active gene transcription.

It is remarkable that in almost all known cases of insertional mutagenesis, retroviruses have inserted at the 5′ end of a given gene, most frequently into the first intron. A Mo-MuLV proviral copy was found in the "intron" of the Rous sarcoma virus (RSV) genome in two revertants of RSV-transformed cells (Varmus *et al.*, 1981). Likewise, a provirus copy has mutated the *p53* gene (Wolf and Rotter, 1984), the *IgG* gene (Kuff *et al.*, 1983), and the β-microglobulin gene (Frankel *et al.*, 1985) by insertion into sequences at the 5′ end of the respective gene. Insertional mutation of the *hprt* gene involved insertion of a Mo-MuLV provirus into an intron in the body of this gene (King *et al.*, 1985). Furthermore, the provirus that caused the *dilute* mutation has integrated into noncoding sequences (Hutchison *et al.*, 1984). It thus appears that proviral copies of spontaneously induced mutations most frequently cluster at the 5′ end of the affected gene, which may suggest that retroviruses do not randomly integrate but have a preference for chromosomal regions with an open chromatin conformation. Recent experiments indeed indicate that all six of the proviral genomes analyzed that are carried in the germ line of Mov substrains or in tissue-culture cells have inserted within 500 base pairs of the next DNase-I-hypersensitive site (Rodewohld *et al.*, 1986).

The high rate of mutations induced in transgenic mice by microinjection of recombinant DNA into the zygote as opposed to retrovirus infection (Table II) deserves comment. The site of integration of the foreign DNA has been analyzed for two lethal mutations induced by the insertion of a human growth-hormone gene (Covarrubias *et al.*, 1985) and for a dysmorphogenetic mutation induced by an M-MTV-myc DNA construct (Woychik *et al.*, 1985). In all three cases, insertation of the multiple copies of the foreign DNA induced rearrangements or deletions or both, at the site of integration. In the two early embryonic lethal mutations, extensive rearrangements of the host sequences flanking the inserted genes have occurred, while the M-MTV-myc integration was associated with a 1-kilobase deletion of sequences flanking the insert. These results suggest that recombinant DNA introduced into transgenic mice by pronuclear injection not only may cause damage by disrupting host sequences at the site of insertion, but also may induce extensive DNA rearrangements in the host genome at other positions, possibly causing second-site mutations. This may complicate or even prevent the isolation of a gene that has been mutated by injection of recombinant DNA. In contrast, no DNA rearrangements have been observed in any of nine analyzed proviral insertions carried in Mov substrains of mice.

Insertional mutagenesis provides a powerful tool for dissecting the genetic mechanisms of mammalian development. The two methods of inducing mutations, infection with retroviruses and pronuclear injection with recombinant DNA, may be mutagenic by different molecular mechanisms. The understanding of these mechanisms will be of importance for evaluating the advantages and disadvantages of the two alternative methods.

ACKNOWLEDGMENTS. This work was supported by Grants HD-19105 from the NIH and PO1-CA 38497 from the National Cancer Institute.

References

Breindl, M., Harbers, K., and Jaenisch, R., 1984, Retrovirus-induced lethal mutation in collagen I gene of mice is associated with altered chromatin structure, *Cell* **38**:9–16.

Covarrubias, L., Nishida, Y., and Mintz, B., 1985, Early developmental mutations due to DNA rearrangements in transgenic mouse embryos, *Cold Spring Harbor Symp. Quant. Biol.* **50**:447–452.

Frankel, W., Potter, T. A., Naomi, R., Lenz, J., and Rajan, T. V., 1985, Retroviral insertional mutagenesis of a target allele in a heterozygous murine cell line, *Genetics* **82**:6600–6604.

Gautsch, J. W., and Wilson, M. C., 1983, Delayed *de novo* methylation in teratocarcinoma suggests additional tissue-specific mechanisms for controlling gene expression, *Nature (London)* **301**:32–37.

Harbers, K., Schnieke, H., Stuhlmann, D., Jähner, D., and Jaenisch, R., 1981, DNA methylation and gene expression: Endogenous retroviral genome becomes infectious after molecular cloning, *Proc. Natl. Acad. Sci. U.S.A.* **78**:7609–7613.

Harbers, K., Kuehn, M., Delius, H., and Jaenisch, R., 1984, Insertion of retrovirus into the first intron of alpha 1(I) collagen gene leads to embryonic lethal mutation in mice, *Proc. Natl. Acad. Sci. U.S.A.* **81**:1504–1508.

Hartung, S., Jaenisch, R., and Breindl, M., 1986, Retrovirus insertion inactivates mouse $\alpha 1$(I) collagen by blocking initiation of transcription, *Nature (London)* **320**:365–367.

Hutchinson, K., Copeland, N., and Jenkins, N., 1984, Dilute coat-colour locus of mice: Nucleotide sequence analysis of the d$^+$-2j and d$^+$-HA revertant allele, *Mol. Cell. Biol.* **4**:2899–2904.

Jaenisch, R., 1976, Germ line integration and Mendelian transmission of the exogenous Moloney leukemia virus, *Proc. Natl. Acad. Sci. U.S.A.* **73**:1260–1264.

Jaenisch, R., 1980, Retroviruses and embryogenesis: Microinjection of Moloney leukemia virus into midgestation mouse embryos, *Cell* **19**:181–188.

Jaenisch, R., and Jähner, D., 1984, Methylation, expression and chromosomal position of genes in mammals, *Biochim. Biophys. Acta* **782**:1–9.

Jaenisch, R., Jähner, D., Nobis, P., Simon, I., Löhler, J., Harbers, K., and Grotkopp, D., 1981, Chromosomal position and activation of retroviral genomes inserted into the germ line of mice, *Cell* **24**:519–529.

Jaenisch, R., Harbers, K., Schnieke, A., Löhler, I., Chumakov, D., Jähner, D., Grotkopp, D., and Hoffman, E., 1983, Germline integration of Moloney murine leukemia virus at the Mov13 locus leads to recessive lethal mutation and early embryonic death, *Cell* **32**:209–216.

Jaenisch, R., Schnieke, A., and Harbers, K., 1985a, Treatment of mice with 5-azacytidine efficiently activates silent retroviral genomes in different tissues, *Proc. Natl. Acad. Sci. U.S.A.* **82**:1451–1455.

Jaenisch, R., Breindl, M., Harbers, K., Jähner, D., and Löhler, J., 1985b, Retroviruses and insertional mutagenesis, *Cold Spring Harbor Symp. Quant. Biol.* **50**:439–445.

Jähner, D., and Jaenisch, R., 1980, Integration of Moloney leukemia virus into the germ line of mice: Correlation between site of integration and virus activation, *Nature (London)* **287**:456–458.

Jähner, D., and Jaenisch, R., 1985a, Chromomosomal position and specific demethylation in enhancer sequences of germ line-transmitted retroviral genomes during mouse development, *Mol. Cell Biol.* **5**:221–222.

Jähner, D., and Jaenisch, R., 1985b, Retrovirus induced *de novo* methylation of flanking host sequences correlates with gene inactivity, *Nature (London)* **315**:594–597.

Jähner, D., Stuhlmann, H., Stewart, C. L., Harbers, K., Löhler, J., Simon, I., and Jaenisch, R., 1982, *De novo* methylation and expression of retroviral genomes during mouse embryogenesis, *Nature (London)* **298**:623–628.

Jenkins, N. A., Copeland, N. G., Taylor, B. A., and Lee, B. K., 1981, Dilute (d) coat color mutation of DBA/2J mice is associated with the site of integration of an ecotropic MuLV genome, *Nature (London)* **293**:370–374.

King, W., Patel, M. D., Lobel, L. I., Goff, S. P., and Nguyen-Huu, M. C., 1985, Insertion mutagenesis of embryonal carcinoma cells by retroviruses, *Science* **228**:554–558.

Kuff, E. L., Feenstra, A., Lueders, K., Smith, L., Hawley, R., Hozumi, N., and Shulman, M., 1983, Intracisternal A-particle genes as movable elements in the mouse genome, *Proc. Natl. Acad. Sci. U.S.A.* **80**:1992–1996.

Löhler, J., Timpl, R., and Jaenisch, R., 1984, Embryonic lethal mutation in mouse collagen I gene causes rupture of blood vessels and is associated with erythropoietic and mesenchymal cell death, *Cell* **38**:597–607.

Mark, W. H., Signorelli, K., and Lacy, E., 1985, An insertional mutation in a transgenic mouse line results in developmental arrest at day 5 of gestation, *Cold Spring Harbor Symp. Quant. Biol.* **50**:453–463.

Palmiter, R. D., Wilkie, T. M., Chen, H. Y., and Brinster, R. I., 1984, Transmission distortion and mosaicism in an unusual transgenic mouse pedigree, *Cell* **36**:869–877.

Reik, W., Weiher, H., and Jaenisch, R., 1985, Replication-competent Moloney murine leukemia virus carrying a bacterial suppressor tRNA gene: Selective cloning of proviral and flanking host sequences, *Proc. Natl. Acad. Sci. U.S.A.* **82**:1141–1145.

Rodewohld, H., Weiher, H., Jaenisch, R., and Breidel, M., 1986, Retrovirus integration and chromatin structure: Moloney Murine Leukemia proviral integration map near DNAse I hypersensitive site, *J. Virol.* (submitted).

Schnieke, A., Harbers, K., and Jaenisch, R., 1983, Embryonic lethal mutation in mice induced by retrovirus insertion into the alpha 1(I) collagen gene, *Nature (London)* **304**:315–320.

Soriano, P., and Jaenisch, R., 1986, Retroviruses as probes for mammalian development: Allocation of cells to the somatic and germ cell lineages, *Cell* **46**:19–29.

Stewart, C. L., Stuhlmann, H., Jähner, D., and Jaenisch, R., 1982, *De novo* methylation, expression, and infectivity of retroviral genomes introduced into embryonal carcinoma cells, *Proc. Natl. Acad. Sci. U.S.A.* **79**:4098–4102.

Stuhlmann, H., Jähner, D., and Jaenisch, R., 1981, Infectivity and methylation of retroviral genomes is correlated with expression in the animal, *Cell* **26**:221–232.

Varmus, H. E., Quintrell, N., and Ortiz, S., 1981, Retroviruses as mutagens: Insertion and excision of a nontransforming provirus alter expression of a resident transforming provirus, *Cell* **25**:23–36.

Wagner, E. F., Covarrubias, L., Stewart, T. A., and Mintz, B., 1983, Prenatal lethalities in mice homozygous for human growth hormone gene sequences integrated in the germ line, *Cell* **35**:647–655.

Wolf, D., and Rotter, V., 1984, Inactivation of p53 gene expression by an insertion of Moloney murine leukemia virus-like sequences, *Mol. Cell. Biol.* **4**:1402–1410.

Woychik, R. P., Stewart, T. A., Davis, L. G., D'Eustachio, P., and Leder, P., 1985, An inherited limb deformity created by insertional mutagenesis in a transgenic mouse, *Nature (London)* **318**:36–40.

11

P Transposable Elements and Their Use as Vectors for Gene Transfer in Drosophila

GERALD M. RUBIN, FRANK A. LASKI, and DONALD C. RIO

1. Introduction

Transposable elements are segments of DNA that move as discrete units from place to place in the genome. They have been found in bacteria, fungi, plants, and animals. The frequency at which these elements move depends on a variety of poorly understood factors including element structure, genetic background, and environmental influences. Transposable elements can comprise a substantial fraction of an organism's genome. For example, approximately 5% of the *Drosophila melanogaster* genome consists of transposable elements. More than 20 different transposable element families have been identified in *D. melanogaster*, and these fall into four structural classes (Rubin, 1983).

P elements, the family of transposable elements that are the causative agents of P–M hybrid dysgenesis in *D. melanogaster*, have been studied intensively, in large part because their mobility can be controlled in the laboratory by manipulating the genetic background of their host (for reviews, see Engels, 1983; Bregliano and Kidwell, 1983). When the elements are quiescent, they are said to be in the *P cytotype* (Engels, 1979a), the cellular environment of P-strain flies. The P cytotype is apparently determined by P elements themselves (Engels, 1979b, 1983).

Flies lacking functional P elements are called *M-strain* flies and are said to possess the *M cytotype*. Hybrid dysgenesis occurs when P-strain

GERALD M. RUBIN, FRANK A. LASKI, and DONALD C. RIO • Department of Biochemistry, University of California, Berkeley, California 94720.

males are crossed with M-strain females, thereby introducing functional P elements into the M cytotype. The offspring of such a cross show a series of genetic aberrations, all of which are confined to the germ lines of these dysgenic hybrids. These aberrations may include chromosomal rearrangements, visible and lethal mutations, male recombination, and a high level of gonadal sterility. In the reciprocal cross, between an M-strain male and a P-strain female, or in P × P cross, the P elements are maintained in the P cytotype, and no dysgenic traits are observed.

A number of P elements have been isolated (Rubin *et al.*, 1982) and characterized (O'Hare and Rubin, 1983). About one third of the 50 elements found in a typical strain share a conserved 2.9-kilobase (kb) structure; the others are heterogeneous in size and are smaller, missing sequences internal to the 31-base-pair terminal inverted repeats that flank the element. The 2.9-kb element has been shown to supply a *trans*-acting function required both for its own transposition (Spradling and Rubin, 1982) and for the transposition of defective nonautonomous P elements (Rubin and Spradling, 1982).

The strategy for using P elements as vectors for gene transfer is based on mimicking the events that take place during a dysgenic cross between P and M strains. In such a cross, P elements on paternally contributed chromosomes enter the M-cytotype egg and are induced to transpose at high rates. An analogous situation occurs if DNA containing a 2.9-kb P element is microinjected into an M-cytotype embryo shortly after fertilization. This element can transpose from the injected DNA to the germline chromosomes of the host embryo in a reaction that is catalyzed by a protein encoded by the P element. Smaller P elements that lack the DNA sequences encode this protein can also transpose if coinjected with the 2.9-kb element. Other DNA segments of interest can be transferred to the germ line if they are inserted within such internally deleted P elements and then coinjected with the 2.9-kb element.

P elements are highly effective vectors for gene transfer. Since genes transferred using P element vectors are incorporated into the germ lines of their hosts, their function can be assayed in all cell types and developmental stages in subsequent generations. Although the transferred genes are not inserted at their normal chromosomal locations, they appear to be regulated properly and, in nearly all cases, exhibit correct tissue and temporal specificity of expression.

2. Results and Discussion

2.1. A Strategy for the Analysis of P-Element Functions

To genetically dissect the functions encoded by P elements, one must be able to examine a single element of defined structure, rather than the heterogeneous population of 2.9-kb and deleted P elements found in the genomes of natural P strains. In addition to its ability to produce the symptoms of hybrid dysgenesis, the element needs to be genetically marked, so that its presence and location in the genome of a living fly can be detected. By inserting the *rosy* gene, which encodes the enzyme xanthine dehydrogenase, into a nonessential region of a 2.9-kb P element, we were able to make a marked P-element derivative that acts in most respects like the unmodified 2.9-kb P element (Karess and Rubin, 1984). When introduced into an M-strain fly, this element, called Pc[*ry*], continues to transpose autonomously within the genome and is able to destabilize other nonautonomous P elements. Our strategy has been to mutagenize the Pc[*ry*] element *in vitro* and assay its activity *in vivo*, both singly and in combination with other P elements, to identify the regions of the element that encode the transposase.

2.2. All Four P-Element Open Reading Frames Are Required for Transposase Activity

The most sensitive assay of P transposase activity involves measuring the rate of destabilization of the *singed weak* (*sn^w*) mutation (Engels, 1984). The *sn^w* is a hypermutable allelle of the *singed bristle* locus on the X chromosome. It arose in the offspring of a dysgenic hybrid (Engels, 1979a), and its phenotype results from the presence of two small, nonautonomous P elements at the *sn* locus that appear to form a head-to-head inverted repeat (H. Roiha, K. O'Hare, and G. Rubin, in prep.). In the offspring of a P male × M female dysgenic cross in which one parent carries *sn^w*, up to 50% of the gametes of the F_1 dysgenic hybrids no longer carry the parental *sn^w* allele (Engels, 1979a, 1984). One or the other of the two nonautonomous P elements at *sn^w* excises, generating one of two new phenotypes in the F_2 offspring: a much more extreme singed bristle (*sn^e*) or an apparently wide-type bristle (*sn^+*) (H. Roiha, K.

O'Hare, and G. Rubin, in prep.). However, the sn^w allelle is essentially stable when it is maintained in a genome devoid of autonomous P elements. Thus the destabilization of sn^w is an extremely sensitive assay for the presence of transposase activity provided by functional P elements. A single autonomous P element is sufficient to induce sn^w instability (Spradling and Rubin, 1982).

The wild-type Pc[ry] element can destabilize sn^w, but mutant derivatives of Pc[ry] containing frameshift mutations in any of the four open reading frames (ORFs) cannot (Karess and Rubin, 1984). Furthermore, no complementation is observed between mutations in different ORFs, suggesting that each of the four ORFs contributes to a single polypeptide required for transposition.

2.3. Tissue Specificity of P-Element Transposition

P-element transposition is limited to the germ-line; transposition has not been observed in somatic tissues (for a review, see Engels, 1983). What is the mechanism by which tissue specificity is achieved? The simplest explanation would be that synthesis of the transposase protein is limited to the germ-line. For example, the transcriptional promoter for the transposase gene might be active only in germ-line cells. Alternatively, transposase might be made in all cells, but other proteins or cofactors needed for the transposition reaction might be germ-line limited. As described below, we have been able to demonstrate by a series of *in vitro* mutagenesis experiments that transposase production is apparently limited to the germ line by a novel mechanism: A germ-line-specific RNA-splicing event is required.

We first asked whether the limitation of transposition to the germ-line could be overcome by substituting a transcriptional promoter known to be highly active in somatic cells for the natural P promoter. P-element constructs that contained the P-element coding sequences were made under the control of the heat-inducible hsp70 promoter (Lis *et al.*, 1983). Although a high level of transcription was observed in somatic cells following heat induction, transposition was still limited to the germ line (Laski *et al.*, 1986).

A clue to the mechanism of germ line specificity is provided by the structure of the major P-element transcript. As described above, the results of *in vitro* mutagenesis experiments suggest that the four ORFs present in the 2.9-kb element are joined by RNA splicing into a single continuous sequence that encodes transposase. Examination of the P-element DNA sequence (O'Hare and Rubin, 1983) reveals that potential 5' and 3' splice sites (Mount, 1982) are indeed located in appropriate positions near the ends of the ORFs. An analysis of the major P-element transcript, however, indicates that the intron postulated to join ORFs 2 and 3 is still present in the mature polyadenylated transcript isolated from embryos and other sources (Laski *et al.*, 1986).

The presence of this intron was puzzling in two respects: First, while there are many examples of differential or alternative RNA-splicing patterns, no case has been reported of a stable RNA in which some, but not all, of the introns have been removed. Second, given that the sequences of ORF 3 are required (Karess and Rubin, 1984), such a transcript should be incapable of encoding active transposase. A way to reconcile this apparent contradiction is to propose that the RNA the structure of which we have analyzed is not in fact a functional messenger RNA (mRNA) for transposase. We isolated RNA from whole embryos in which only about 1% of the cells are of the germ-line lineage. Perhaps removal of the ORF 2–ORF 3 intron, and thus the production of functional transposase mRNA, occurs only in the germ line. Given the very low abundance of P transcripts (Karess and Rubin, 1984), such a small fraction of fully spliced RNA might have escaped our detection.

We tested the hypothesis that germ line-specific splicing of the ORF 2–ORF 3 intron is the basis for the tissue specificity of transposase production by constructing a number of Pc[*ry*] elements in which this intron was either removed or altered (Laski *et al.*, 1986). These elements were introduced into *Drosophila* and assayed for *sn*^w destabilization as described by Karess and Rubin (1984).

Consistent with the hypothesis that removal of the intron is a prerequisite for transposase production, mutations that alter the consensus 5' or 3' splice sites of this last intron abolish transposase production as assayed by *sn*^w destabilization. The mutation that proved to be most informative was one that removed the intron, thereby joining the coding sequences of ORFs 2 and 3 without the need for RNA splicing. Flies carrying such a mutant element, which we call Pc[*ry*,Δ2-3], produce in their germ lines as much transposase as, if not more transposase than, do those with wild-type Pc[*ry*] elements. Most important, however, they now produce transposase in their somatic cells as well. This can be seen most easily by the ability of Pc[ry,Δ2-3] elements to induce somatic mosaicism by causing transposition and excision of P elements in somatic cells.

Two assays were used to detect somatic transposase activity. In the first assay, which measures somatic P-element excision, flies carrying a Pc[ry,Δ2-3] element are crossed with flies carrying a nonautonomous transposon, P[w^+], as their only normal copy of the *white* locus. Such flies have red eyes by virtue of the wild-type *white* gene contained within the P[w^+] transposon. The F_1 offspring of such a cross will carry both the P[w^+] and the Pc[ry,Δ2-3] element. Autonomous P elements, such as Pc[ry], are able to induce the excision of nonautonomous elements, such as P[w^+]. Normally, this activity is limited to the germ line, and in such a case all the F_1 offspring would have red eyes, as only their germ lines would be mosaic. Since the *white* gene is cell-autonomous, somatic excisions of P[w^+] would produce clones of nonpigmented cells in the eye. Such clones are observed in early all flies carrying both the P[w^+] and the Pc[ry,Δ2-3] transposon.

The second assay is designed to measure transposition of a P[w^+] element from one chromosome site to another. In this assay, the P[w^+] transposon used confers a pale yellow eye color due to its location at a site in the genome that precludes normal *white* gene expression (Hazelrigg *et al.*, 1984). Transposition of this P[w^+] to a new genomic site or transposase-induced local rearrangements can each restore a red eye color (Levis *et al.*, 1985). Evidence of such somatic events, which produce red clones on the yellow background, are seen in the eyes of nearly all flies carrying both this P[w^+] transposon and the Pc[ry,Δ2-3] element. The size and number of clones observed suggest that multiple events occur in the cell lineage leading to each eye and that these events can occur both early and late in development.

2.4. P-Element-Encoded Proteins

We have identified proteins encoded by P transposable elements expressed in transformed *Drosophila* tissue-culture cells (Rio *et al.*, 1986). Two proteins have been identified by immunochemical techniques. One, an 87,000-dalton polypeptide, is encoded by a P-element mRNA lacking the third (ORF 2–ORF 3) intervening sequence. The other protein, a 66,000-dalton polypeptide, is encoded by an mRNA that retains the third intron and is found in somatic tissues. Furthermore, tissue-culture cell lines that express the 87,000-dalton polypeptide are able to catalyze both the precise and the imprecise excision of a nonautonomous P element. As would be expected from the results of the *in vitro* mutagenesis experiments described above, immunochemical data indicate that the 87,000-dalton putative transposase is encoded by sequences from all four P-element ORFs (Rio *et al.*, 1986).

Taken together, our data strongly suggest that the sole basis for the limitation of P-element transposition to the germ line is the failure to remove a particular intron from P transcripts in somatic cells. Further experiments will be required to determine whether germ line-specific RNA splicing is used to control the expression of other genes or is peculiar to P elements. In addition to these biological questions, the ability to induce somatic mosaics at high frequency may be useful in marking cells for lineage studies. Moreover, it is possible that removal of the intron between ORFs 2 and 3 will not only overcome the germ line limitation but also broaden the host range of P-element transposition to include other organisms. Preliminary results using the plasmid-excision assay suggest that functional P-element transposase can be expressed in cultured mammalian cells.

References

Bregliano, J. C., and Kidwell, M. G., 1983, Hybrid dysgenesis determinants, in: *Mobile Genetic Elements* (J. A. Shapiro, ed.), Academic Press, New York, pp. 363–410.

Engels, W. R., 1979a, Extrachromosomal control of mutability in *Drosophila melanogaster, Proc. Natl. Acad. Sci. U.S.A.* **76**:4011–4015.

Engels, W. R., 1979b, Hybrid dysgenesis in *Drosophila melanogaster:* Rules of inheritance of female sterility, *Genet. Res.* **33**:219–236.

Engels, W. R., 1983, The P family of transposable elements in *Drosophila, Annu. Rev. Genet.* **17**:315–344.

Engels, W. R., 1984, A *trans*-acting product needed for P factor transposition in *Drosophila, Science* **226**:1194–1196.

Hazelrigg, T., Levis, R., and Rubin, G. M., 1984, Transformation of *white* locus DNA in *Drosophila:* Dosage compensation, *zeste* interaction, and position effects, *Cell* **36**:469–481.

Karess, R. E., and Rubin, G. M., 1984, Analysis of P transposable element functions in *Drosophila, Cell* **38**:135–146.

Laski, F. A., Rio, D. C., and Rubin, G. M., 1986, The tissue specificity of *Drosophila* P element transposition is regulated at the level of mRNA splicing, *Cell* **44**:7–19.

Levis, R., Hazelrigg, T., and Rubin, G. M., 1985, Effects of genomic position on the expression of transduced copies of the *white* gene of *Drosophila, Science* **229**:558–561.

Lis, J. T., Simon, J. A., and Sutton, C. A., 1983, New heat shock puffs and β-galactosidase activity resulting from transformation of *Drosophila* with an *hsp70-lacZ* hybrid gene, *Cell* **35:**403–410.

Mount, S. M., 1982, A catalog of splice junction sequences, *Nucleic Acids Res.* **10:**459–472.

O'Hare, K., and Rubin, G. M., 1983, Structures of p transposable elements and their sites of insertion and excision in the *Drosophila melanogaster* genome, *Cell* **34:**25–35.

Rio, D. C., Laski, F. A., and Rubin, G. M., 1986, Identification and immunochemical analysis of biologically active *Drosophila* P element transposase, *Cell* **44:**21–32.

Rubin, G. M., 1983, Dispersed repetitive DNAs in *Drosophila*, in: *Mobile Genetic Elements* (J. A. Shapiro, ed.), Academic Press, New York, pp. 329–362.

Rubin, G. M., and Spradling, A. C., 1982, Genetic transformation of *Drosophila* with transposable element vectors, *Science* **218:**348–353.

Rubin, G. M., Kidwell, M. G., and Bingham, P. M., 1982, The molecular basis of P–M hybrid dysgenesis: The nature of induced mutations, *Cell* **29:**987–994.

Spradling, A. C., and Rubin, G. M., 1982, Transposition of cloned P elements into *Drosophila* germ line chromosome, *Science* **218:**341–347.

12

Mapping and Manipulating Immunoglobulin Functions

MARC J. SHULMAN

1. Introduction

Nature is comprised of a multitude of organisms, all of us competing for a finite supply of nutrients. But for our immune system, which functions to recognize and eliminate foreign substances, we would ourselves be excellent culture media for many of the faster-growing organisms.

Immunoglobulin (Ig) molecules serve as a soluble receptor for the immune system. As such, Ig accomplishes two tasks: (1) binding specifically to foreign material of diverse structures (2) delivering it for treatment by the immune system. This bipartite function is reflected in the structural organization of the Ig molecule. The variable (V) region of the Ig molecule can have many different amino acid sequences, and this variability allows the production of binding sites of diverse specificities. The other part of the Ig molecule, the constant (C) region, has relatively few amino acid sequences and is responsible for interacting with the effector mechanisms of the immune system.

Specific Ig's will probably have diverse applications, both in therapy and as preparative and diagnostic reagents. Our understanding of Ig biosynthesis and Ig structure and function is probably adequate for designing effective reagents. However, the features of Ig that are important in human therapy are still poorly defined. We do not know, for example, which structural features of which C regions influence the therapeutic ef-

MARC J. SHULMAN • Department of Immunology, University of Toronto, Toronto, Ontario, Canada M5S 1A8.

fectiveness of specific Ig. This chapter will review the available technology for producing Ig and the way in which Ig structure can be manipulated to engineer more effective molecules. It will also present some results of our ongoing work, which we hope will more precisely define the molecular requirements of Ig biosynthesis and function.

2. Immunoglobulin Gene and Protein Structure

The basic Ig monomer unit contains two identical heavy (H) chains (≈ 450–575 amino acids) and two identical light (L) chains (≈ 220 amino acids) (Fig. 1). The chains are held together both by disulfide bonds and by noncovalent interactions. The H and L chains fold into distinct domains of approximately 110 amino acids. These domains, whether from the V or C region or the H or L chain, have some structural features in common. For example, the general domain structure can be represented as two β-pleated sheets, one three-stranded and one four-stranded, with the apposition of the two sheets stabilized by disulfide bonds (Fig. 2). The individual domains differ in important structural features that determine their distinctive functions. The amino-terminal domains of the H and L

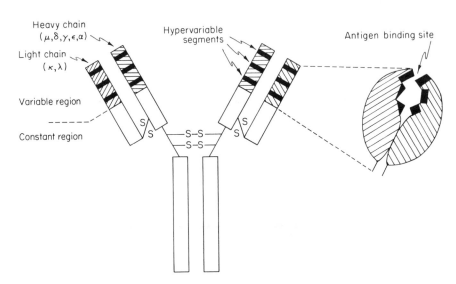

Figure 1. Schematic diagram of Ig structure.

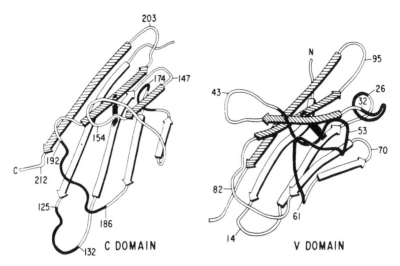

Figure 2. Secondary structure of Ig light chain domains. The structure of an Ig domain includes two antiparallel β-pleated sheets. The three-chain β-sheet is indicated by the striated arrows, the four-chain sheet by white arrows. The carboxy (C) and amino (N) termini are marked. The numbers indicate amino acid positions. Chain segments that are present in only one domain or that have different structures in the two domains are shown as solid black lines. From Edmundson *et al.* (1975).

chains together compose the V region; these domains bind in such a way that their three-stranded sheets are juxtaposed. By contrast, the interaction of the C-region domains of the H and L chains juxtaposes their four-stranded sheets, and this arrangement is stabilized by an intermolecular disulfide bond. The μ and α chains have at their carboxy terminus an extra segment of 20 amino acids that mediates their assembly into pentameric IgM and multimeric IgA (reviewed in Beale and Feinstein, 1976; Burton, 1985; Koshland, 1985).

The chains are named according to the amino acid sequence of their C region. Thus, L chains are of two general types, λ and *x*, while H chains (and the corresponding Ig's) are of five general types, μ (IgM), δ (IgD), γ (IgG), α (IgA), ε (IgE). The conventional nomenclature denotes Ig composed of μ and *x* chains as IgM(*x*), of γ and λ chains as IgG(λ), and so on. The manner in which the Ig interacts with the immune system is thought to depend on the H-chain C region. For example, IgM and some subtypes of IgG can mediate complement-dependent lysis of their target cells, and the binding of the complement component C1 depends on residues in the third C domain of the μ chain (see below) and the second C domain of the γ chain (reviewed in Burton, 1985). Some subtypes of IgG, but not of IgM, can mediate the action of killer cells in antibody-dependent cellular cytotoxicity (ADCC). The specific binding of Ig to viruses or bacteria enhances their engulfment by macrophages, and the interaction with macrophages apparently depends on both the second and third C domains of IgG.

As mentioned above, an individual organism—mouse or man—can produce many distinct Ig V regions. By contrast, an individual Ig-producing cell expresses only one V region; i.e., the great diversity in the Ig repertoire reflects the great heterogeneity among Ig-producing cells. The molecular basis for this heterogeneity was predicted by Dreyer and Bennett (1965) and is outlined in Fig. 3. The DNA segment that encodes the Ig H and L chains is assembled in somatic cells into functional genes, illustrated in the figure for the H chain. Within the genome are approximately 100 V segments that encode the first 95 amino acids of the V domain, approximately 12 diversity (D) segments that encode the next few amino acids, and approximately 4 joining (J) segments that encode the final 13 amino acids of the V domain.

During ontogeny, potential Ig-producing cells join one V, one D, and one J segment to construct a functional H-chain gene. If all combinations of V, D, and J segments could be joined to give a functional V region, this mechanism could generate approximately 5000 different amino acid sequences. The joining of the segments is often accompanied by the insertion or deletion of several nucleotides at the junction, thus increasing the number of possible V-region sequences. Further diversity can arise as mutations occur during the proliferation of antibody-producing cells (see below). A similar process involving only V and J segments is used to construct an L-chain gene. Thus, this mechanism is expected to generate more than 10^7 distinct combinations of H- and L-chain V-region domains. In ways yet to be completely defined, the cell contrives to make only one functional rearrangement for the H and L chain per cell and thus can express only one V region (reviewed by Tonegawa, 1983).

The genetic structure shown in the second line of Fig. 3 would encode a μ (or δ) H chain. The expression of the μ and δ genes seems to be determined by differential RNA transcription or processing (Maki *et al.*, 1981; Moore *et al.*, 1981)—perhaps by messenger RNA cleavage or polyadenylic acid addition, or both, as seems to be the case for the differential expression of the μ-chain membrane and secreted forms (Dan-

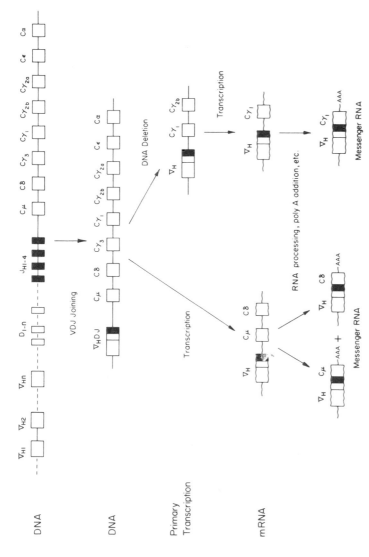

Figure 3. Rearrangement of DNA to generate a functional H-chain gene. The top line shows the germ-line arrangement of genes for the mouse Ig H-chains. Exons are indicated as boxes, to distinguish them from the noncoding introns and flanking sequences. The second line depicts the DNA structure following the rearrangements that construct a functional V region. This DNA can be transcribed into RNA (wavy lines) as shown or undergo further rearrangements to juxtapose the functional V with another H-chain C region.

ner and Leder, 1985). In a process known as the *class switch*, the cell manages to express the V region with other H-chain C regions. In cell lines that express C regions downstsream of δ, the DNA that encodes the intervening C regions has been deleted; e.g., the μ-δ-γ C regions are deleted in cell lines that produce the α H chain. Such results have suggested that deletion is the mechanism for the switch to these H-chain classes, although two groups have adduced evidence that in some cell types, γ, ϵ, and α H-chain expression might also be controlled by differential RNA processing (Yaoita *et al.*, 1982; Perlmutter and Gilbert, 1984).

Burnet (1959) devised the clonal selection theory to explain the specificity of the immune response (Fig. 4). Many cells, each capable of making Ig of different specificity, lie dormant in the organism, with Ig situated as a receptor on their membrane. Part of the signal for proliferation occurs when antigen interacts with the membrane Ig. Thus, the cells making Ig that binds the antigen are specifically stimulated to divide. Furthermore, mutants in which the V region is altered and antigen is better bound are expected to outgrow cells making the original Ig. In practical terms, these features mean that a properly immunized animal will nearly always manage to generate cells making Ig that is highly specific for the immunizing antigen.

The typical antigen presents several different "foreign determinants," each of which can elicit an immune response. Furthermore, an animal is capable of making multiple distinct Ig's that react with an individual determinant. The cells that proliferate in response to the antigen are thus heterogeneous (polyclonal) themselves. With present technololgy, the lifetime of these normal Ig-producing cells is finite, even in the presence of antigen, thus limiting the amount of Ig that can be made by normal cells. Another technical problem in making Ig with normal cells is that different clones predominate in different animals, even when the animals are genetically identical. These considerations mean that it is very difficult or even impossible to obtain the same spectrum of Ig's from two individuals.

3. Production of Monoclonal Immunoglobulins from Mouse and Man

The hybridoma technique devised by Kohler and Milstein (1975) overcomes the problems described above by providing a way of immortaliz-

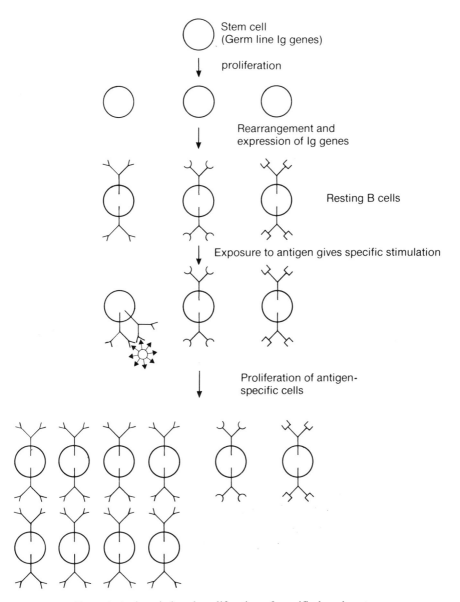

Figure 4. Antigen-induced proliferation of specific lymphocytes.

ing and cloning the Ig-producing cells (Fig. 5). The first step in this procedure is the immunization of the mouse to increase the frequency of antigen-specific Ig-producing cells. These cells, usually obtained from the mouse spleen, are then fused with an immortal myeloma-tumor-cell line. This procedure generates a hybridoma that has inherited the capacity for eternal growth from the tumor parent and the properly rearranged H- and L-chain genes from the normal Ig-producing cell. While it can be difficult to locate and clone out the hybridoma that is producing specific Ig, this method seems to yield a general solution to the antibody-production problem by providing an unlimited amount of homogeneous Ig of virtually any specificity.

While the mouse is in many cases the best available animal for making specific Ig-producing hybridoma-cell lines, we can anticipate circumstances in which humans might be a better source. For example, it might be easier to obtain cells making Ig specific for transplantation or blood-group antigens from exposed individuals. It appears that the hybridoma system can be used with human cells, although the technology is at present less reliable than for mouse cells. Different laboratories use different tumor-cell fusion partners and procedures to generate specific cell lines (reviewed in Cole *et al.*, 1985). Two groups in particular have reported successful

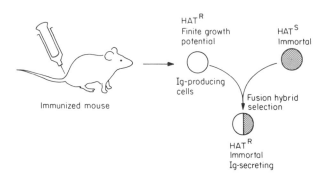

Figure 5. Generation of hybridoma cell lines. Normal spleen cells from an immunized mouse are fused with (immortal) myeloma cells. The formation of hybrid cells is rare, and to select them, the method uses myeloma cells that bear a mutation in the gene for hypoxanthine phosphoribosyltransferase (HPRT) and are therefore unable to grow in hypoxanthine–aminopterin–thymidine (HAT) medium. The normal spleen cells have a functional *hprt* gene but are incapable of sustained growth in ordinary medium. The hybrid inherits both HPRT$^+$ from the spleen-cell parent and immortality from the myeloma parent and unlike the parent cells can therefore grow indefinitely in HAT medium.

hybridoma production using hybrid human–mouse myelomas as the fusion partner (Teng *et al.*, 1983; Foung *et al.*, 1984). Human peripheral-blood cells can often be used to make hybridomas, so that making human hybridomas can be done without excising the spleen. Furthermore, it is possible to use Epstein–Barr virus rather than fusion with tumor cells to immortalize human Ig-producing cells (reviewed in Roome and Reading, 1984). In summary, the technology for making specific human Ig-producing cell lines is moderately good. Because important ethical considerations restrict the immunization step, the limiting factor is probably the availability of individuals who have been adventitiously immunized in an appropriate way. Even this limitation might be overcome in the future if the immunization of cells *in vitro* can be improved.

4. Uses of Specific Immunoglobulins

For many applications, we need be concerned only with the Ig V region. For example, when the Ig is to be used to purify an antigen, detect virus in blood, or type bacteria, the H- or L-chain C region is usually not important. When Ig is to be used in therapy, on the other hand, it might be very important to use Ig that bears the appropriate C region, as well as the specific V region.

We envision using Ig for therapy in two general ways. The first is as an antibody in the conventional sense: Ig's that are specific for the virus envelope or for bacterial surface antigens could be administered to protect infected individuals. Such Ig would be expected to mobilize the effector mechanisms of the immune system much as though the Ig were produced *in vivo*. In more ambitious scenarios, Ig specific for a tumor-associated antigen could be used to direct the immune system against tumor cells. In such cases, protection might depend on such phenomena as ADCC or complement-dependent cytolysis and therefore might be strongly dependent on the H-chain C region (for studies of the potential importance of the C region in therapy, see Kaminski *et al.*, 1986; Lefrancois, 1984). One alternative to mobilizing the natural effector mechanisms of the patient's immune system is to couple toxic factors (e.g., ricin or radioactive compounds) to specific Ig, which is then expected to target the toxicity appropriately (reviewed in Sikora *et al.*, 1984; Vitetta and Uhr, 1985). Several groups have proposed constructing bifunctional antibodies—cross-linking two antibodies of different specificities to generate Ig that could bind cytotoxic T cells and could also bind specific targets (Staerz *et al.*, 1985; Liu *et al.*, 1986). In such a bridging, the bifunctional Ig can direct nonspecific cytotoxic cells against any cell for which there is a specific Ig.

The other general application for specific Ig might be as an *antigen* for use as a vaccine (reviewed in Bona and Moran, 1985; Kohler *et al.*, 1985). Although some vaccines will be made using recombinant DNA to produce antigenic proteins for vaccination, some important antigens will be made of nonprotein material, such as oligosaccharides, that cannot be so easily produced using recombinant DNA technology. An alternate approach uses the specific V region of Ig in place of the antigen (Fig. 6). Ig specific for the relevant antigen is made using the mouse hybridoma method. The V region of this specific Ig can then be used to immunize another mouse to obtain hybridomas making Ig that is specific for this V region (antiidiotypic Ig). As illustrated in Fig. 6, some of these antiidiotypic Ig's are expected to share structural features with the original antigen and can be used for immunization in place of the original antigen. Here, too, we would expect that the immunization might depend on the H-chain C region. For example, the "wrong" C region might specifically mobilize the ADCC system to kill the cells that were otherwise destined to produce specific Ig.

5. Optimizing Immunoglobulin Structure for Therapy

The species from which Ig is derived may prove to be an important consideration. For example, human Ig might function better in human therapy than mouse Ig of the same specificity. One reason is that the C regions of human and mouse Ig's may interact differently with human effector mechanisms. In addition, the immune system of the patient is expected to see only the V region of human Ig as a potential antigen, whereas mouse Ig presents antigens in both the V and the C region. Patients treated with mouse Ig make anti-Ig directed predominantly against the C region and the anti-Ig appears to interfere with therapy (Meeker *et al.*, 1985).

Genetic engineering enables us to optimize the V and C regions separately. Since the technology for this approach has been published (Boulianne *et al.*, 1984; Morrison *et al.*, 1984; Neuberger *et al.*, 1984), and its application to real therapy is in progress in many laboratories, only the major points will be summarized here.

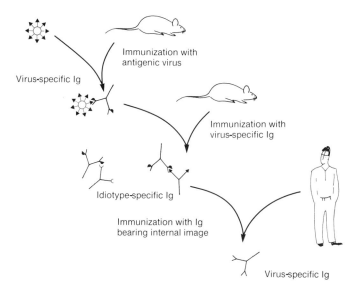

Figure 6. Generation of antiidiotypic antibodies for use as vaccines.

Consider the hypothetical situation in which the only way to get specific antiviral Ig is to make mouse hybridomas and in which specific Ig with the human γ1 C region works best for human antiviral therapy. Under such circumstances, it might be best to produce "chimeric" Ig, in which the V domains of the specific mouse Ig are joined to the human γ1 and L-chain C regions. The organization of the Ig genes facilitates the construction of recombinant DNA that encodes such chimeric Ig (Fig.7). That is, the DNAs that encode the V and C domains are separated by a large intron, so that the corresponding DNAs can be easily isolated and ligated in the combinations desired. These chimeric genes can then be inserted into vectors for transfer into an appropriate tumor-cell line, where they can be expressed to produce chimeric mouse–human Ig bearing the appropriate specificity.

In summary, it is likely that specific Ig's will have wide-ranging therapeutic applications. The major importance of hybridoma/genetic engineering technology today is that it can be used to make Ig with V region of virtually any predefined specificity, which can be expressed with any C region. For the first time, it will be possible to test the usefulness of Ig in therapy in a systematic way. It might, in fact, be possible to domesticate the immune system.

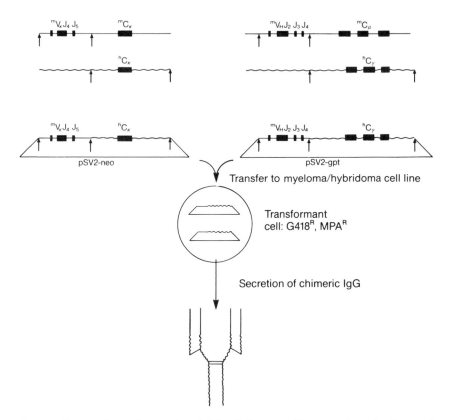

Figure 7. Construction and expression of chimeric Ig genes. The genes for antigenic-specific mouse (superscript m) H and L chains are isolated from a mouse hybridoma-cell line. Using appropriate restriction enzymes to introduce cuts (↑) flanking the exons for the V and C regions, chimeric genes are constructed by joining mouse V-region genes to human (superscript h) C-region genes. These chimeric genes are inserted into transfer vectors and used to transform appropriate (e.g., myeloma) cells. Transformants then express the chimeric genes as the corresponding chimeric Ig, i.e., a mouse V region fused to a human C region. Here, two transfer vectors are illustrated: pSV2-neo, which confers resistance to the drug G418 (Southern and Berg, 1982), and pSV2-gpt, which confers resistance to mycophenolic acid (MPA) (Mulligan and Berg, 1981).

6. Identifying the Molecular Requirements for Immunoglobulin Synthesis and Function

It might be useful to extend the genetic engineering approach to produce Ig's with unprecendented features, such as novel combinations of functions. Some part of the ϵ H chain is required to stimulate mast cells; some feature of the α H chain promotes polymerization; some site of the μ H chain is needed to activate complement. If we wish to produce Ig's in which these functions are altered or made in new combinations, we must first know in detail which amino acid residues are important for Ig function. This is a large undertaking and will require different approaches. Our own work in this area will be described here.

IgM normally contains five disulfide-linked monomeric Ig units. Pentameric IgM forms a star-shaped molecule and includes one J protein as well as the ten H and ten L chains. In mouse IgM, the inter-μ chain disulfide bonds are at Cys337, in the second C domain, and at Cys575, the penultimate amino acid of the μ chain (Milstein *et al.*, 1975). The classic pathway for complement-dependent cytolysis is initiated when the latent protease of the first complement component, C1, is activated by its interaction with Ig (reviewed in Cooper, 1985). A single molecule of pentameric IgM bound to the cell surface can apparently activate C1 (Borsos and Rapp, 1965). The inability of free IgM molecules in solution to activate C1 has suggested that the C1-binding site on IgM is normally unavailable but is exposed when the IgM is distorted by multivalent binding, such as to a cell surface or to large molecules (Borsos and Rapp, 1965; Brown and Koshland, 1975). To activate C1, therefore, IgM must be multimeric (e.g., pentameric), have appropriate affinity for cell-surface antigen, and have a normal C1-binding site.

One method of deducing the function of particular sites of the μ H chain would be to engineer specific alterations in the μ gene and measure the properties of the IgM that bears the corresponding abnormal μ chain. We have taken the converse approach by selecting mutant hybridoma-cell lines that produce noncytolytic IgM and then ascertaining the corresponding mutations that have occurred in the mutant μ genes (Kohler and Shulman, 1980; Shulman *et al.*, 1982). Hybridoma cells present the Ig genes in a way that makes this approach unusually easy. Since hybridomas usually have only one copy of the Ig genes per cell, recessive mutations have a readily detectable phenotype. We have also developed efficient methods of selecting and screening rare mutant cells that produce abnormal IgM.

The starting point for this project is a hybridoma that secretes hapten-specific IgM, and for this purpose we have used two haptens, phosphoryl-choline (Shulman *et al.*, 1982) and trinitrophenyl (Kohler and Shulman, 1980). We mutagenized the wild-type hybridoma-cell line and then exposed it to a reactive derivative of the hapten that couples covalently to the surface membrane of the hybridoma cells. As a cell secretes the hapten-specific IgM, that IgM binds preferentially to the hapten on the surface of that cell. In the presence of complement, the normal cells are lysed, whereas mutants that make less IgM or noncytolytic IgM are spared. Each application of this procedure gives a 10- to 100-fold enrichment for mutants. By growing out the survivors and repeating the procedure a few times, we obtain a population that contains only mutant cells. The cells are then plated out at limiting dilution, and thereafter we measure culture supernatant for the amounts of IgM and its cytolytic titer. From this ratio, we can deduce whether the mutant makes abnormal IgM (structural mutant) or a reduced amount of normal IgM (regulatory mutant). When the mutants make abnormal IgM, we classify that IgM with various tests to evaluate hapten binding, pentamer formation, and gross structure of the μ and $\varkappa$ chains.

Mutants making IgM that does not activate complement were of two general types. The first type was a series of mutants that make monomeric rather than pentameric IgM. These are expected to be useful for defining the molecular requirements for pentamer formation. Two other mutants, denoted No. 13 and No. 42, represent the second type: They make pentameric IgM with normal hapten binding that is nevertheless noncytolytic. The IgM of these mutants is less able to bind C1 (F. Wright, personal communication). These mutants can therefore serve to indicate residues that are important in the interaction between C1 and IgM.

We have recently ascertained the nucleotide change in mutant No. 42. For this purpose, we isolated the DNA that encodes mutant No. 42 μ-chain C region. We assayed this segment for the mutation by incorporating it into a μ-gene transfer vector and expressing it in a mutant hybridoma-cell line that has lost the μ gene but continues to produce the hapten specific $\varkappa$ gene. The IgM made after gene transfer of the recombinant μ gene was defective in its ability to lyse haptenated cells. We then further localized the mutation by constructing recombinant genes bearing various segments from the normal and mutant $C\mu$ genes. The nucleotide sequence results revealed a single base change such that in the mutant μ chain, asparagine replaces serine at amino acid position 406 in the third C region ($C\mu3$) domain. Crystallographic analyses of various Ig's indicate that the structures of the individual domains are in large part independent of each other and therefore suggest that effects of these substitutions on protein secondary structure might be restricted to the $C\mu3$ domain. These results suggest that the secondary structure of the $C\mu3$ domain is important for complement activation.

Other workers have implicated various parts of the IgM molecule in complement activation. Hurst *et al.* (1975) found that a fragment of the fourth C domain of the μ chain could bind and activate the C1 component, albeit at low efficiency. Siegel and Cathou (1981) argued that complement activation could be influenced by the second C domain of the μ H chain. Leptin and Melchers (1982) found that a nonclonal antibody that binds to Cμ3 blocks complement-dependent lysis, whereas antibodies against the other three C domains do not, suggesting that a site in Cμ3 is important for complement activation.

Analysis of the interactions of IgG and complement leads us to expect that the Cμ3 domain is involved in C1 activation. The second C domain of the γ H chain (Cγ2) is thought to be analogous to the Cμ3 domain (Putman *et al.*, 1973), and studies using fragments of IgG molecules have suggested a role for the Cγ2 doman in complement binding and activation (Colomb and Porter, 1975; Yasmeen *et al.*, 1976). Further evidence implicating Cγ2 is the decreased activity of deglycosylated IgG: IgG is glycosylated only at Asn297 in the Cγ2 domain, and deglycosylated IgGs of various types and species are less able to activate complement than is normal IgG (Koide *et al.*, 1977; Winkelhake *et al.*, 1980; Nose and Wigzell, 1983; Leatherbarrow *et al.*, 1985). In the context of a model in which the Ig domains are structurally independent, these results suggest that C1 activation depends on the structure of the Cγ2 domain and thus, by extension, on the structure of the Cμ3 domain.

The μ chain of mutant No. 42 appears to be abnormally glycosylated. That is, when the μ chains are unglycosylated (synthesized in the presence of tunicamycin), the wild-type and mutant chains comigrate; however, the glycosylated mutant μ chain migrates more slowly than the glycosylated normal μ chain (Shulman *et al.*, 1982). Glycosylation occurs at asparagine residues in the sequence Asn-X-Ser/Thr (Hubbard and Ivatt, 1981). The change Ser406 $\rightarrow$ Asn generates the sequence Asn-Ala-Lys, which is not expected to be a site for glycosylation. The migration of the mutant μ chain thus raises the interesting possibility that the amino acid substitution influences the glycosylation at another Asn. For example, glycosylation in Cμ3 normally occurs at Asn402 and Asn364 (Kehry *et al.*, 1979), and the Ser406 $\rightarrow$ Asn change might alter the pattern of glycosylation of these nearby oligosaccharides. Another possibility is that the Asn-Phe-Thr sequence at positions 347–349, which is not normally glycosylated (Kehry *et al.*, 1979), has become a substrate for glycosylation in the mutant No. 42 μ chain.

Taken together, these results suggest that the Ser406 $\rightarrow$ Asn change might affect the interaction of IgM and complement by altering the glycosylation of the μ chain. If so, this mutant would offer an unusual opportunity to analyze the way in which the amino acid sequence of the IgM protein influences the specificity of glycosylation and how, in turn, the oligosaccharide structure can influence protein function.

We have also examined mutant No. 102, which makes monomeric IgM (Baker *et al.*, 1986). To define this mutation, we made a complementary DNA (cDNA) corresponding to the μ-chain RNA of mutant No. 102. The nucleotide sequence of this cDNA was identical to the wild-type except that it lacked 39 base pairs corresponding to amino acids 550–562. We have introduced this deletion into the normal μ gene and verified that it generates monomeric IgM like that of the original mutant. The results of Rogers *et al.* (1980) concerning the splicing of the Cμ4 and membrane exons suggest that the boundary of the Cμ4 exon is at amino acid 556 and that the tail comprises the last 20 amino acids. The deletion thus removes 7 amino acids of the fourth C doman (Cμ4) and 6 of the tail, a region previously postulated to be involved in pentamer formation. The remaining 14 amino acids, including Cys575, which would normally be used to bind μ chains into the pentamer, are presumably present.

7. Future Studies on the Structural and Regulatory Mutants

The mutants that we have isolated give us an entry into several areas of research. We can use them as a starting point for *in vitro* site-directed mutagenesis to obtain a systematic and extensive analysis of related sites in the μ H chain. One unanticipated result has been that many of the mutants appear to glycosylate their μ chains abnormally (Shulman *et al.*, 1982) and *cis/trans* tests indicate that this phenotype reflects mutations in the μ gene (M. Yoshimura, personal communication). Previous work by many investigators has shown that the structure of the oligosaccharides on glycoproteins is specified partly by the various glycosidases and glycosyltransferases and partly by the structure of the substrate protein (reviewed by Hubbard and Ivatt, 1981). These mutants therefore offer the opportunity to correlate precisely how changes in amino acid sequence can affect glycosylation. Similarly, the regulatory mutants can serve to identify the sites in the gene that are important for gene expression.

However, we suspect for a number of reasons that our current gene-transfer and mapping technology will prove inadequate for studying regulatory mutants. For example, the gene-transfer techniques that we now use yield transformants that themselves differ greatly in level of gene expression. Furthermore, the effect of the mutations on gene expression may depend on chromosomal context (site of integration), or it may be due to changes, such as methylation, that are not preserved when the genes are produced in bacteria. Another problem is that the mutations might map outside the DNA segment that we clone and assay. In the analysis of microbial (yeast, bacterial, or phage) mutants, these problems are avoided, because mutations can be mapped by the frequency of homologous recombination (e.g., recombination between transferred DNA and the resident genome). Several groups have shown that a similar form of homologous recombination occurs in mammalian cells in tissue culture (Smithies *et al.*, 1985; Lin *et al.*, 1985; Thomas *et al.*, 1986). If these recombination studies can be developed into a method for mapping mutations in the Ig gene, the mutations can then serve to reveal molecular requirements for gene expression that would otherwise be unrecognizable.

References

Baker, M. D., Wu, G. E., Toone, W. M., Murialdo, H., Davis, A. C., and Shulman, M. J., 1986, A region of the immunoglobulin μ heavy chain necessary for forming pentameric IgM, *J. Immunol.* **137**:1724–1728.

Beale, D., and Feinstein, A., 1976, Structure and function of the constant regions of immunoglobulins, *Q. Rev. Biophys.* **9**:135–171.

Blattner, F. R., and Tucker, P. W., 1984, The molecular biology of immunoglobulin D, *Nature (London)* **307**:417–422.

Bona, C., and Moran, T., 1985, Idiotype vaccines, *Ann. Inst. Pasteur Immunol.* **136**:299–312.

Borsos, T., and Rapp, H. J., 1965, Complement fixation on cell surfaces by 7S and 19S antibodies, *Science* **150**:505–506.

Boulianne, G. L., Hozumi, N., and Shulman, M. J., 1984, Production of functional chimeric mouse/human antibody, *Nature (London)* **312**:643–646.

Brown, J. C., and Koshland, M. E., 1975, Activation of antibody Fc function by antigen-induced conformational changes, *Proc. Natl. Acad. Sci. U.S.A.* **72**:5111–5115.

Burnet, F. M., 1959, *The Clonal Selection Theory of Acquired Immunity*, Cambridge University Press, London.

Burton, D. R. 1985, Immunoglobulin G: Functional sites, *Mol. Immunol.* **22**:161–206.

Cole, S. P. C., Kozbor, D., and Roder, J. C. C., 1985, Strategies for production of human monoclonal antibodies, in: *Hybridoma Technology in the Biosciences and Medicine* (T. A. Springer, ed.), Plenum Press, New York, pp. 43–55.

Colomb, M., Porter, R. R., 1975, Characterization of a plasmin-digest fragment of rabbit immunoglobulin gamma that binds antigen and complement, *Biochem. J.* **145**:177–183.

Cooper, N. R., 1985, The classical complement pathway: Activation and regulation of the first complement component, *Adv. Immunol.* **37**:151–216.

Danner, D., and Leder, P., 1985, Role of an RNA cleavage/poly (A) addition site in the production of membrane-bound and secreted IgM RNA, *Proc. Natl. Acad. Sci. U.S.A.* **82**:8658–8662.

Dreyer, W. J., and Bennett, J. C., 1965, The molecular basis of antibody formation: A paradox, *Proc. Natl. Acad. Sci. U.S.A.* **54**:864.

Edmundson, A. B., Ely, K. R., Abola, E. E., Schiffer, M., and Panagiotopoulos, N., 1975, Rotational allomerism and divergent evolution of domains in immunoglobulin light chains, *Biochemistry* **14**:3953–3961.

Foung, S. K. H., Perkins, S., Raubitschek, A., Larrick, J., Lizak, G., Fishwald, D., Engelman, E. G., and Grummet, F. C., 1984, Rescue of human monoclonal antibody production from an EBV-transformed B cell line by fusion to a human–mouse hybridoma, *J. Immunol. Methods* **70**:83–90.

Hubbard, S. C., and Ivatt, R. J., 1981, Synthesis and processing of asparagine-linked oligosaccharides, *Annu. Rev. Biochem.* **50**:555–583.

Hurst, M. M., Volanakis, J. E., Stroud, R. M., and Bennett, J. C., 1975, C1 fixation and classical component pathway activation by a fragment of the $C\mu 4$ domain of IgM, *J. Exp. Med.* **142**:1322–1326.

Kaminski, M. S., Kitamura, K., Maloney, D. G., Campbell, M. J., and Levy, R., 1986, Importance of antibody isotype in monoclonal anti-idiotype therapy of a murine B cell lymphoma: A study of hybridoma class switch variants, *J. Immunol.* **136**:1123–1130.

Kehry, M., Sibley, C., Fuhrman, J., Schilling, J., and Hood, L. E., 1979, Amino acid sequence of a mouse immunoglobulin μ chain, *Proc. Natl. Acad. Sci. U.S.A.* **76**:2932–2936.

Kohler, G., and Milstein, C., 1975, Continuous cultures of fused cells secreting antibody of predefined specificity, *Nature (London)* **256**:495–497.

Kohler, G., and Shulman, M. J., 1980, Immunoglobulin M mutants, *Eur. J. Immunol.* **10**:467–476.

Kohler, H., Muller, S., and Bona, C., 1985, Internal antigen and immune network, *Proc. Soc. Exp. Biol. Med.* **178**:189–195.

Koide, N., Nose, M., and Muramatsu, T., 1977, Recognition of IgG by Fc receptor and complement: Effects of glycosidase digestion, *Biochem. Biophys. Res. Commun.* **75**:838–844.

Koshland, M. E., 1985, The coming of age of the immunoglobulin J chain, *Annu. Rev. Immunol.* **3**:425–453.

Leatherbarrow, R. J., Rademacher, T. W., Dwek, R. A., Woof, J. M., Clark, A., Burton, D. P., Richardson, N., and Feinstein, A., 1985, Effector functions of a monoclonal aglycosylated mouse IgG2a: Binding and activation of complement component C1 and interaction with human monocyte Fc receptor, *Mol. Immunol.* **22**:407–415.

Lefrancois, L., 1984, Protection against lethal viral infection by neutralizing and non-neutralizing monoclonal antibodies: Distinct mechanisms of action *in vivo, J. Immunol.* **51**:208–214.

Leptin, M., and Melchers, F., 1982, A monoclonal antibody with specificity for mouse μ heavy chain which inhibits the formation of antigen-specific direct IgM plaques, *J. Immunol. Methods* **59**:53–61.

Lin, F. L., Sperle, K., and Sternberg, N., 1985, Recombination in mouse L cells between DNA introduced into cells and homologous chromosomal sequences, *Proc. Natl. Acad. Sci. U.S.A.* **82**:1391–1395.

Liu, M. A., Kranz, D. M., Kurnick, J. T., Boyle, L. A., Levy, R., and Eisen, H. N., 1986, Heteroantibody duplexes target cells for lysis by cytotoxic T lymphocytes, *Proc. Natl. Acad. Sci. U.S.A.* **82**:8648–8652.

Maki, R., Roeder, W., Traunecker, A., Sidman, C., Wabl, M., Raschke, W., and Tonegawa, S., 1981, The role of DNA rearrangement and alternative RNA processing in the expression of immunoglobulin delta genes, *Cell* **24**:353–365.

Meeker, T. C., Lowder, J., Maloney, D. G., Miller, R. A., Theilemans, K., Warnke, R., and Levy, R., 1985, A clinical trial of anti-idiotype therapy for B cell malignancy, *Blood* **65**:1349–1363.

Milstein, C. P., Richardson, N. E., Deverson, E. V., and Feinstein, A., 1975, Interchain disulphide bridges of mouse immunoglobulin M, *Biochem. J.* **151**:615–624.

Moore, K. W., Rogers, S., Hunkapillar, T., Early, P., Nottenburg, C., Weissman, I., Bazin, H., Wall, R., and Hood, L. E., 1981, Expression of IgD may use both DNA rearrangement of RNA splicing mechanisms, *Proc. Natl. Acad. Sci. U.S.A.* **78**:1800–1804.

Morrison, S. L., Johnson, M. J., Herzenberg, L. A., and Oi, V. T., 1984, Chimeric human anitbody molecules: Mouse antigen-binding domains with human constant region domains, *Proc. Natl. Acad. Sci. U.S.A.* **81**:6851–6858.

Mulligan, R. C., and Berg, P., 1981, Selection for animal cells that express the *Escherichia coli* gene coding for xanthine-guanine phosphoribosyl transferase, *Proc. Natl. Acad. Sci. U.S.A.* **78**:2072–2076.

Neuberger, M. S., Williams, G. T., and Fox, R. O., 1984, Recombinant antibodies possessing novel effector functions, *Nature (London)* **312**:604–608.

Nose, M., and Wigzell, H., 1983, Biological significance of carbohydrate chains on monoclonal antibodies, *Proc. Natl. Acad. Sci. U.S.A.* **80**:6632–6636.

Perlmutter, A. P., and Gilbert, W., 1984, Antibodies of the secondary response can be expressed without switch recombination in normal mouse B cells, *Proc. Natl. Acad. Sci. U.S.A.* **81**:7189–7193.

Putnam, F. W., Florent, G., Paul, C., Shinodo, T., and Shimizu, A., 1973, Complete amino acid sequence of the mu heavy chain of a human IgM immunoglobulin, *Science* **182**:287–291.

Rogers, J., Early, P., Carter, C., Calame, K., Bond, M., Hood, L., and Wall, R., 1980, Two mRNAs with different 3′ ends encode membrane-bound and secreted forms of the immunoglobulin μ chain, *Cell* **20**:303–312.

Roome, A. J., and Reading, C. L., 1984, The use of Epstein–Barr virus transformation for the production of human monoclonal antibodies, *Exp. Biol.* **43**:35–55.

Shulman, M. J., Heusser, C., Filkin, C., and Kohler, G., 1982, Mutations affecting the structure and function of immunoglobulin M, *Mol. Cell. Biol.* **2**:1033–1043.

Siegel, R. C., and Cathou, R. E., 1981, Effects of limited denaturation by heat on the dynamic conformation of equine immunoglobulin M antibody and on interaction with antigen and complement, *Biochemistry* **20**:192–198.

Sikora, K., Smedley, H., and Thorpe, P., 1984, Tumour imaging and drug targeting, *Br. Med. Bull.* **40**:233–239.

Smithies, O., Gregg, R. G. Boggs, S. S., Koralewski, M. A., and Kucherlapti, R. S., 1985, Insertion of DNA sequences into the human chromosomal β-globin locus by homologous recombination, *Nature (London)* **317**:230–234.

Southern, P. J., and Berg, P., 1982, Transformation of mammalian cells to antibiotic resistance with a bacterial gene under the control of SV40 early region promoter, *J Mol. Appl. Genet.* **1**:327–241.

Staerz, U. D., Kanagawa, O., and Bevan, M. J., 1985, Hybrid antibodies can target sites for attack by T cells, *Nature (London)* **314**:628–631.

Teng, N. N. H., Lam, K. S., Riera, F. C., and Kaplan, H. S., 1983, Construction and testing of mouse–human heteromyelomas for human monoclonal antibody production, *Proc. Natl. Acad. Sci. U.S.A.* **80**:7308–7312.

Thomas, K. R., Folger, K. R., and Cappechi, M. R., 1986, High frequency targeting of genes of specific sites in the mammalian genome, *Cell* **44**:419–428.

Tonegawa, S., 1983, Somatic generation of antibody diversity, *Nature (London)* **302**:575–581.

Vitetta, E. S., and Uhr, J. W., 1985, Immunotoxins, *Annu. Rev. Immunol.* **3**:197–212.

Winkelhake, J. L., Kunicki, T. J., Elcombe, B. M., and Aster, R. H., 1980, The effects of pH treatments and deglycosylation of rabbit immunoglobulin G on the binding of C19, *J. Biol. Chem.* **255**:2822–2828.

Yaoita, Y., Kumewgai, Y., Okumura, K., and Honjo, T., 1982, Expression of lymphocyte surface IgE does not require switch recombination, *Nature (London)* **297**:697–699.

Yasmeen, D., Ellerson, J. R., Dorrington, K. J., and Painter, R. H., 1976, The structure and function of immunoglobulin domain. IV. The distribution of some effector functions among the Cγ2 and Cγ1 homology regions of human immunoglobulin G, *J. Immunol.* **116**:504–509.

13

T4: A T-Cell Surface Protein Mediating Cell–Cell and Cell–AIDS Virus Interactions

ANGUS G. DALGLEISH, PAUL J. MADDON,
DAN R. LITTMAN, PAUL R. CLAPHAM,
MAURICE GODFREY, LEONARD CHESS, ROBIN A. WEISS,
J. STEVEN McDOUGAL, and RICHARD AXEL

1. Introduction

The different functional classes of T lymphocytes recognize antigen on the surface of distinct populations of target cells. Helper T cells interact largely with macrophages and B cells; cytotoxic T cells interact with a broader range of antigen-bearing target cells. These cellular recognition events are likely to be mediated by the specific association of surface molecules on both effector and target cells. The surface of T cells is characterized by a number of polymorphic, as well as nonpolymorphic, proteins that are restricted for the most part to T lymphocytes. Although most of these molecules are common to all T cells, two classes of surface proteins consistently differ on the different functional classes of ma-

ANGUS G. DALGLEISH, PAUL R. CLAPHAM, and ROBIN A. WEISS • Institute of Cancer Research, Chester Beatty Laboratories, London SW3 6JB, England.   PAUL J. MADDON • Department of Biochemistry and Molecular Biophysics, College of Physicians and Surgeons, Columbia University, New York, New York 10032.   MAURICE GODFREY and LEONARD CHESS • Department of Medicine, College of Physicians and Surgeons, Columbia University, New York, New York 10032.   J. STEVEN McDOUGAL • Immunology Branch, Centers for Disease Control, Atlanta, Georgia 30333.   DAN R. LITTMAN and RICHARD AXEL • Howard Hughes Medical Institute, College of Physicians and Surgeons, Columbia University, New York, New York 10032.

ture T lymphocytes: the T-cell antigen receptor and the surface glycoproteins T4 and T8. These proteins have therefore been implicated in T cell–target cell interactions.

In the peripheral immune system, the T4 and T8 molecules are expressed on mutually exclusive subsets of T lymphocytes and are only rarely expressed on the same cell (Reinherz and Schlossman, 1980; Blue *et al.*, 1985). The T4 molecule is expressed on T cells that interact with targets that bear class II major histocompatibility complex (MHC) proteins, whereas T8-bearing T cells interact with targets that express class I MHC proteins (Engleman *et al.*, 1981a; Krensky *et al.*, 1982; Meuer *et al.*, 1982; Biddison *et al.*, 1982; Wilde *et al.*, 1983; Swain, 1983). The T4$^+$ population of T lymphocytes contains helper T cells, whereas the T8$^+$ population contains the majority of cytotoxic and suppressor T cells (Thomas *et al.*, 1981; Meuer *et al.*, 1982). However, rare T4$^+$ T lymphocytes can function as cytotoxic or suppressor cells (Thomas *et al.*, 1981, Meuer *et al.*, 1982), suggesting that the expression of T4 or T8 is associated more stringently with MHC class recognition than with effector function.

The significance of these molecules in T cell–target cell interactions can be demonstrated by studies with monoclonal antibodies. Antibodies directed against specific epitopes of the T4 molecule (or the murine equivalent, L3T4) inhibit antigen-induced T-cell proliferation, lymphokine release, and helper-cell function (Engleman *et al.*, 1981b; Biddson *et al.*, 1982; Wilde *et al.*, 1983; Marrack *et al.*, 1983; Rogozinski *et al.*, 1984). Similarly, monoclonal antibodies directed against T8 (or the murine equivalent, Lyt2) inhibit cytotoxic-T-cell-mediated killing (Swain, 1981; Landegren *et al.*, 1982). These observations, along with the fact that T4 and T8 do not reveal significant polymorphism, have led to the hypothesis that T4 and T8 recognize nonpolymorphic regions of class II and class I proteins, respectively. In this manner, T4 and T8 may be responsible for the specific targeting of functionally distinct populations of T lymphocytes. More recently, evidence has accumulated to suggest that T4 may serve not only as a receptor for molecules on the surface of target cells, but also as a receptor of a T lymphotropic retrovirus, the acquired immune deficiency syndrome (AIDS) virus (Dalgleish *et al.*, 1984; Klatzmann *et al.*, 1984b; McDougal *et al.*, 1986).

We have combined the procedures of gene transfer and subtractive hybridization to isolate the complementary DNAs (cDNAs) and genes that encode the T-cell surface glyoproteins T4 and T8 (Maddon *et al.*, 1985; Littman *et al.*, 1985). The protein sequences of T4 and T8 reveal N-terminal extracellular domains with amino acid and structural homologies to the variable (V) region of immunoglobulin light (L) chains. The protein sequences and predicted molecular structures are consistent with the hypothesis that these molecules function as recognition elements on the T-cell surface. Moreover, genetic and biochemical experiments demonstrate that the T4 glycoprotein is a receptor for the AIDS virus, and the mere presence of T4 on the cell surface is sufficient to render a variety of human cell types susceptible to AIDS virus infection.

2. Results

2.1. Isolation of Complementary DNAs That Encode Both T4 and T8

The experimental approach we used to isolate the T4 and T8 genes initially involved gene transfer to generate mouse L-cell contransformants that expressed either the T4 or T8 glycoprotein on their surface. Complementary DNA synthesized from the messenger RNA (mRNA) of these transformants was hybridized to a vast excess of mRNA from nontransformed L cells, generating a cDNA probe highly enriched for those sequences introduced into the L cell by gene transfer. This probe was used to screen a library of cDNA clones prepared from the mRNA of human peripheral T lymphocytes. The identities of cDNA clones obtained in this manner were verified by several independent experiments (Littman *et al.*, 1985; Maddon *et al.*, 1985). First, Northern-blot analyses were performed to determine the pattern of expression of RNA encoded by the cDNA clones. A putative T4 cDNA detects a 3-kilobase (kb) mRNA present in the T4$^+$ transformant that is also present in a population of T4$^+$ peripheral T lymphocytes, several T4$^+$ leukemic T-cell lines, and thymocytes. No hybridization is observed with RNA from untransformed fibroblasts, T4$^-$ peripheral T lymphocytes, or several T4$^-$ human cell lines. Similarly, a putative T8 clone hybridizes to a 2.4-kb mRNA with a pattern of expression that is consistent with its identity as T8. Second, Southern-blot experiments were performed that demonstrate that sequences homologous to either the T4 or T8 clones are present in human DNA as well as in T4$^+$ or T8$^+$ transformed mouse L cells, but not in untransformed mouse L-cell DNA. Third, full-length cDNAs that encode T4 and T8 were introduced into eukaryotic expression vectors. These DNA constructs were then used to convert mouse fibroblasts to either the T4$^+$ or the T8$^+$ phenotype following infection or transformation. Finally, in the case of T8, a partial N-terminal sequence has recently been provided (Snow *et al.*, 1984) that is encoded by our T8 clone.

2.2. Nucleotide Sequences of T4 and T8

We have determined the complete nucleotide sequences of the T4 and T8 coding regions by sequencing both strands of the cDNA inserts using the dideoxy termination procedure. The deduced protein sequences reveal that both molecules are comprised of a hydrophobic signal sequence, a variable or V-like domain, a second extracellular region, a hydrophobic membrane-spanning domain, and a highly charged cytoplasmic segment (Fig. 1). Comparison of the protein sequences of T4 and T8 indicates that these molecules share significant sequence and structural homology with immunoglobulin domains and are members of the immunoglobulin supergene family (Fig. 2). However, the N-terminal V-like domains of T4 and T8 are quite different; they share only 28% homology and are

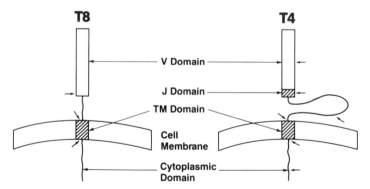

Figure 1. Schematic diagram of the T4 and T8 proteins spanning the cell membrane. Both T4 and T8 are comprised of an extracellular V-like domain, a second extracellular region, a hydrophobic membrane-spanning domain, and a highly charged cytoplasmic segment. In addition, the J-like domain abuts the V-like domain of the T4 molecule. (→) Positions of introns in the corresponding genes. For the complete nucleotide and protein sequences, see Littman *et al.* (1985) and Maddon *et al.* (1985).

therefore less homologous to each other than each is to immunoglobulin L chains. Moreover, the regions of maximum conservation between T4 and T8 are also the regions of strongest homology with immunoglobulin and T-cell antigen-receptor V regions. Thus, the putative receptor domains of these two molecules, although structurally similar, show significant sequence divergence consistent with the hypothesis that they recognize different molecules on different subsets of target cells.

Several additional differences distinguish T4 and T8. The V-like domain of T4 is immediately followed by a block of amino acid residues that has considerable homology with the consensus joining (J) regions of both immunoglobulin L chains and T-cell antigen-receptor chains (Figs. 1 and 2). A similar J-region homology is not evident in T8. The J-like region of T4 is followed by a stretch of 265 amino acids on the extracellular surface that has little apparent homology with members of the immunoglobulin supergene family or to any protein in the NIH protein data base. This region is significantly longer and bears no homology with the comparable 58-amino-acid stretch in T8. As a consequence, T4, which contains 435 amino acids, is about twice the size of T8. In summary, T4 and T8 share overall structural homology: Both molecules are integral membrane proteins with an extracellular domain homologous to an immunoglobulin L-chain V region, a transmembrane segment, and a charged cytoplasmic domain. At the level of amino acid sequence, however, they are very different: Their V-like domains are highly divergent, the proteins differ dramatically in size, and they share a low overall sequence homology.

The V-like region structural homology shared by the N-terminal domains of T4 and T8 may be of particular relevance to the putative function of these proteins. Virtually all members of the immunoglobulin supergene family participate in the immune response (Hood *et al.*, 1985). Moreover, the individual members of this family show a strong tendency to associate with each other to form dimers. This association is apparent in the interaction of the heavy and light chains of immunoglobulin, the α and β chains of the T-cell antigen receptor, β_2-microglobulin and class I MHC proteins, and the α and β chains of class II MHC molecules. The T8 glyoprotein forms a disulfide bond with T6, a presumed MHC-like molecule, on the surface of thymocytes (Snow *et al.*, 1986) and exists as multimers of the 32-kilodalton (kd) subunit on peripheral T lymphocytes (Snow and Terhorst, 1983). These specific affinities of im-

A

```
                    10              20              30              40            50
T4         - - Q G N K V V - - L G K K - I G D T V E L T C T A S Q K K - S I Q F H W K N S N Q I K I L G N Q G S F L T K G P
V-kappa    D V Q M I Q S P S S L S A S L G D I V T M T C Q A S Q G - T S I N W F Q Q K P G K - A P K - - L L I Y G A
Inv.       - S Q F R V S P L D R T W N L G E T V E L K C Q V L L S N P T S G C S W L F Q P R G A A A S P T - - F L L Y L S
T8         D A G V I Q S P R H E V T E M G Q E V T L R C K P I S G - H N S L F W Y R Q T M M R G L E - - L L I Y F N
YT35       - Q K V T Q A Q T E I S V V E K E D V T L D C V Y E T R D T T Y Y L F W Y K Q P P S G E L V - - F L I R R N
HPB-MLTα
               A               B               C               C'
```

```
                    60              70              80              90
T4         - - S K L - - - - N D R A D S R R S L W D Q G N F - P L I H K N L K I E D S D T Y I C E V E D Q K E E - -
V-kappa    - - S I L E - D - - - G V P S - R F S G S R Y G T D - F T L T I S S L Q H S Y L P Y - -
Inv.       Q N K P K A A E - G L D T Q - R F S G K R - L G D T - F V L T L S D F R R E N E G Y F C A L S N S I M - -
T8         N N V P I D D - S G M P E D R F S A K M P N - A S - F S T L K I Q P S E P R D S A V Y F C A S S F S T C S A N - -
YT35       - - S F D E Q N E I S G - - R Y S W N F Q K - S T S S E - N F T I T A S Q V V D S A V Y F C A L D S S A S K - -
HPB-MLTα
               D               E               F               G
```

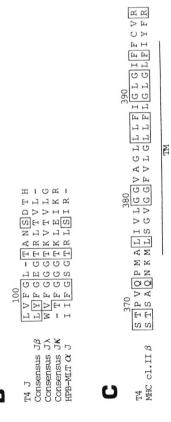

B

```
                        100
T4 J           L V F G L - T A N S D T H
Consensus Jβ   L Y F G E G T R L T V L -
Consensus Jλ   W V F G G G T K V T V L G
Consensus JK   - T F G G G T K L E I K R
HPB-MLT α J    I I F G S G T R L S I R -
```

C

```
              370           380           390
T4           S T P V Q P M A L I V L G G V A G L L L F I G L G I F F C V R
MHC cl.II β  S T S A Q N K M L S G V G G F V L G L L F L G L F I Y F R
                                          TM
```

Figure 2. Alignment of the variable (V) joining (J), and transmembrane regions of T4 with members of the immunoglobulin gene family. (A) Alignment of the V-region amino acid sequence of T4 with a mouse κ L-chain immunoglobulin J606 (Kabat *et al.*, 1983), T8 (Littman *et al.*, 1985), a human T-cell antigen-receptor β chain YT35 (Yanagi *et al.*, 1984), and a human T-cell antigen-receptor α chain HPB-MLTα (Sim *et al.*, 1984). The invariant (Inv.) residues in the L-chain V region are included in the alignment. The alignment was performed to maximize identities and structural homologies with T4, which appear as boxed residues. The horizontal lines below the sequence lettered A, B, C, C′, D, E, F, and G indicate the residues that form β-strands (Williams *et al.*, 1984). β-Strand G continues into the J sequence. (B) Alignment of the J-region amino acid sequence of T4 with the consensus J sequences of the T-cell antigen-receptor β-chain, immunoglobulin λ and κ L chains, and the J sequence of the human T-cell receptor α chain (Saito *et al.*, 1984). (C) Alignment of the transmembrane regions of T4 and an MHC class II β-chain (Saito *et al.*, 1983). The putative transmembrane domain (TM) is indicated below the sequence.

munoglobulinlike molecules may be essential for the putative recognition functions of T4 and T8.

2.3. Evolution of T4 and T8

In the immunoglobulin and T-cell antigen-receptor genes, the V and J exons are widely separated and become juxtaposed only after a somatic recombination event (Tonegawa, 1983; Hood *et al.*, 1985). The T4 mRNA encodes contiguous V- and J-like elements without the requirement for DNA recombination events. It is therefore possible that T4 reflects a more primitive gene that evolved before the emergence of rearrangement mechanisms. Further support for this possibility derives from recent observations from our laboratory (Fig. 1) (P. J. Maddon, D. E. Maddon, and R. Axel, unpublished data) that the V-like region of T4 is split by an intron not present in either the V genes that encode the immunoglobulins or those that encode T-cell antigen receptors. Accumulating evidence suggests that it is far more likely for introns to be precisely removed during evolution than for introns to be inserted in a previously intron-free environment. Thus, T4 may represent an ancestral immunoglobulin gene that underwent duplications, divergence, and rearrangement to generate the current immunoglobulin gene family. Although functional in a far more complex immune system at present, T4 may therefore reflect receptors operative in more primitive cellular immune responses. Primitive immune responses, such as those of invertebrates, do not appear to involve a diverse repertoire of receptor molecules, but in the simplest cases are restricted to a distinction between self and nonself (Hildemann, 1979; Scofield *et al.*, 1982) and are likely to be accommodated by a "static" set of genes that do not undergo rearrangement.

Whatever the order of appearance of T4 and T8 in evolutionary time, the organization of these genes reveals an interesting example of exon shuffling. T4 consists of a V-like domain, a J-like region, and a transmembrane segment, each sharing homology with different members of the immunoglobulin supergene family. The V- and J-like domains are homologous to the equivalent regions of both immunoglobulin and T-cell antigen-receptor chains; the transmembrane domain shows considerable homology with this region in the β-chains of class II MHC molecules (see Fig.2). T4 therefore consists of a collection of exons, conserved in several members of the immunoglobulin supergene family, that are shuffled in different ways to generate a large number of different molecules that participate in the immune response.

2.4. T4 Expression Is Required for AIDS Virus Infection

The T4 molecule may serve not only as a receptor that recognizes molecules on the surface of target cells, but also as a receptor of a T lymphotropic RNA virus. The human acquired immune deficiency syndrome results from the infection of T lymphocytes with a collection of closely related viruses, the AIDS viruses (LAV or HTLV-III) (Barre-Sinoussi *et al.*, 1983; Gallo *et al.*, 1984). The range of infectivity of these agents is restricted to cells that express surface T4 protein (Klatzmann *et al.*, 1984a; Dalgleish *et al.*, 1984). These observations have led to the suggestion that T4 may itself serve as a specific receptor for the AIDS virus. These suggestions have been supported by studies demonstrating that monoclonal antibodies directed against T4 epitopes block AIDS virus infection of T4$^+$ cells (Dalgleish *et al.*, 1984; Klatzmann *et al.*, 1984b). Furthermore, recent studies have demonstrated that when T4$^+$ T lymphocytes are exposed to AIDS virus, the 110-kd envelope glycoprotein of the virus can be coprecipitated with the T4 molecule on the target cell (McDougal *et al.*, 1986). The availability of the T4 cDNA and the ability to introduce T4 into new cellular environments has allowed us to examine the role of the T4 glycoprotein in AIDS virus infection in greater detail.

In an initial series of experiments, we asked whether the presence of the T4 protein on the surface of a lymphocyte is sufficient to render the cell susceptible to AIDS virus infection. To this end, we initially chose a primitive T-cell leukemic line, HSB2, which expresses only the early T-lymphocyte antigens, T1 and T11, on its surface. HSB2 expresses neither T4 nor T8, nor does it express the T-cell receptor or the associated complex of T3 proteins. We have used several different experimental approaches to assess the susceptibility of HSB2 to AIDS virus infection, including syncytium induction (Dalgleish *et al.*, 1984), expression of reverse transcriptase, expression of viral antigens in the cytoplasm of the cell, and detection of virus in the culture supernatant (McDougal *et al.*, 1985). Using these assays, we have not observed evidence for either AIDS virus entry or viral replication in this cell. Thus, The T4$^-$ T-cell line HSB2 cannot support AIDS virus infection.

In addition, we have tested for viral entry using pseudotypes of vesicular stomatitis virus (VSV) bearing the envelope antigens of the AIDS virus (Clapham *et al.*, 1984). When cells infected with AIDS virus are superinfected with VSV, a proportion of the progeny VSVs assemble sufficient envelope glycoprotein of the AIDS virus to resist neutralization by hyperimmune anti-VSV serum. The host range of these VSV(AIDS) pseudotype virions is restricted to cells that express receptors specific to the AIDS virus. Following penetration of the cell and uncoating of the virion, the transcapsidated VSV genome replicates to produce nonpseudotype particles that infect and destroy neighboring cells. Thus, VSV(AIDS) pseudotypes provide a quantitative cytopathic plaque assay for viral entry (Dalgleish *et al.*, 1984). In this assay, no plaques over background are observed when HSB2 cells are exposed to VSV(AIDS) pseudotypes (Table I). Independent experiments with pseudotypes of VSV(HTLV-I) demonstrate that the HSB2 cell is capable of replicating VSV efficiently. These observations demonstrate that the VSV genetic information encapsidated in an AIDS virus envelope is incapable of entering HSB2 cells.

We then asked whether the introduction of a functional T4 gene into HSB2 renders this cell susceptible to AIDS virus infection. We have introduced the T4 cDNA into a retroviral expression vector, pMV7 (P. T. Kirschmeier, G. M. Housey, M. D. Johnson, A. S. Perkins, I. B. Weinstein, unpublished data), that contains two Moloney murine sarcoma virus long terminal repeats (LTRs) as well as the thymidine kinase promoter fused to the coding region of the neomycin phosphotransferase gene (Maddon *et*

Table I. Susceptibility of T4+ and T8+ Cells to AIDS Virus Infection[a]

Human cell	Reverse transcriptase (cpm/ml)	Syncytium induction	Pseudotype infection	Supernate virus	Cytoplasmic virus	Virus binding
CEM (T4+)	675,023	+	+	+	+	+
HSB2	4,245	−	−	−	−	−
HSB2-T8+	4,460	−	−	−	−	−
HSB2-T4+	190,915	+	+	+	+	+
Raji	ND	−	−	ND	ND	ND
Raji-T8+	5,595	−	−	−	−	−
Raji-T4+	103,500	+	+	+	+	+
HeLa	6,438	−	−	−	−	−
HeLa-T8+	4,875	−	ND	−	−	−
HeLa-T4+	48,125	+	+	+	+	+

[a](ND) Not determined.

al., 1985). The 5′ LTR promotes transcription through the inserted T4 cDNA and the 3′ LTR contains sequences necessary for cleavage and polyadenylation. This DNA construct was used to transfect ψ-AM (Cone and Mulligan, 1984), a cell line that produces the viral proteins of an amphotropic retrovirus incapable of packaging its own RNA, but capable of packaging other retroviral RNAs introduced into this cell line. A neomycin-resistant transformant of ψ-AM was selected that produces a recombinant virus that encodes the T4 cDNA encapsidated by an amphotropic viral coat capable of infecting most human cells. When this cell line, ψ-AM T4A, is treated with mitomycin C and cocultivated with HSB2 cells, virtually all T lymphocytes are infected with virus and express a neomycin-resistant phenotype. Flow-cytometry analysis of HSB2-T4$^+$ cells exposed to fluorescein-conjugated anti-T4 antibody demonstrates that virtually all neo$^+$ cells are expressing T4 on their surface (Fig. 3). In a similar manner, we have used retrovirus-mediated gene transfer to introduce T8 into the HSB2 cell line, serving as a control in these studies.

When HSB2-T4$^+$ cells are exposed to VSV(AIDS) pseudotypes, infectious VSV is produced by these cells. Moreover, exposure of HSB2-T4$^+$ cells to intact AIDS virus results in the replication of this virus as determined by syncytium induction, reverse transcription assays, expression of viral antigens in the cytoplasm of the cell, and the production of infectious virus in culture supernatant (Table I). Control HSB2-T8$^+$ cells are consistently negative in each of these assays. These results provide genetic evidence that in an immature T lymphocyte, the mere presence of T4 provides an essential function required for AIDS virus infection.

2.5. Infection by AIDS Is Not Restricted to T Lymphocytes

We next asked whether infection by AIDS virus is restricted to T4$^+$ T lymphocytes or whether the introduction of T4 into nonlymphocytic cell lines will render these cells susceptible to AIDS virus infection. We have introduced the T4 gene into two non-T-cell lines: HeLa, an epithelial cell line derived from cervical carcinoma, and Raji, a B-cell line originally derived from Burkitt's lymphoma. These cell lines do not express T4 mRNA or surface protein, and neither is infectible by AIDS virus or a VSV(AIDS) pseudotype (Table I). Both Raji and HeLa cell lines were then infected with the recombinant retrovirus that encodes the T4 cDNA, and populations of T4$^+$ cells were isolated. T4$^+$ Raji and HeLa cells constructed in this manner support AIDS virus infection (Table I). In addition, exposure of these

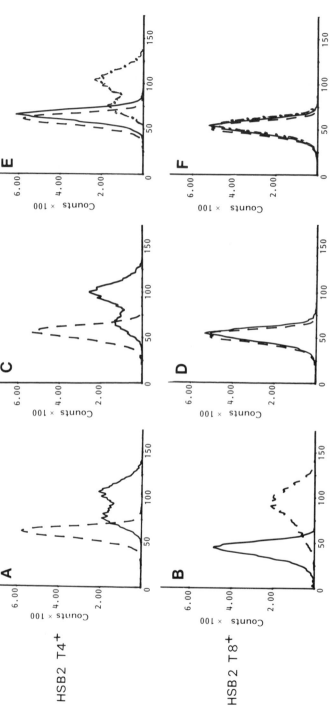

Figure 3. Flow cytometry analysis of the binding of AIDS virus to cells transformed with retroviruses that encode the human T4 or T8 gene. (A, B) Fluorescence histograms (cell number vs. log fluorescence) of HSB2 cells transformed with T4 (A) or T8 (B). The cells were incubated with fluorescein-conjugated anti-T8 (———) or anti-T4A (———) monoclonal antibodies and were then analyzed by flow cytometry. (C, D) HSB2-T4+ cells (C) and HSB2 T8+ cells (D) were incubated with either buffer (———) or AIDS virus (———), followed by fluorescein-conjugated anti-HTLV-III antibodies. (E, F) HSB2-T4+ cells (E) or HSB2-T8+ cells (F) were first incubated with buffer followed by AIDS virus (———), with the monoclonal antibody anti-T4A followed by AIDS virus (———), or with anti-T8 antibody followed by AIDS virus (-•-•-). After washing, fluorescein-conjugated anti-HTLV-III virus antibodies were added, and the cells were then analyzed by cytofluorimetry.

cells to VSV(AIDS) pseudotypes results in the production of infections VSV (Table I). Thus, the expression of surface T4 protein on either human T lymphocytes, B lymphocytes, or epithelial cells is sufficient to render them susceptible to AIDS virus infection. These observations demonstrate that the T4$^+$ T-cell tropism observed *in vivo* is a consequence of the T4 molecule itself and not of the nature of the cell type in which it resides.

2.6. T4 Serves as a Receptor for AIDS Virus

The previous experiments provide genetic evidence that T4 expression is required for AIDS virus infection, but do not provide information on the role of this molecule in the viral life cycle. The observation that surface expression of T4 is required for AIDS virus infection immediately suggests that T4 may be the AIDS virus receptor. We have used cytofluorometry to examine the binding of AIDS virus to the surface of T4$^+$ and T4$^+$ transformants. T4$^-$/T8$^-$ HSB2, Raji, and HeLa cells, and the T4$^+$ or T8$^+$ transformants, were incubated with AIDS virus. Following viral absorption, cells were exposed to fluorescein-conjugated anti-HTLV-III and analyzed by flow cytometry. This assay demonstrates that the AIDS virus binds equally efficiently to the three cell types that express surface T4, but not to the T4$^-$ parental cells or to the T8$^+$ transformants (Fig. 3 and Table I). Moreover, the binding of AIDS virus to T4$^+$ cells is inhibited by preincubation with anti-T4A monoclonal antibody, but not by preincubation with anti-T8 monoclonal anbtibody (Fig. 3). These studies demonstrate that the AIDS virus binds to the T4 molecule on the cell surface and that this binding is likely to be independent of other T-cell-specific proteins, since binding occurs to all T4$^+$ cell types examined.

2.7. Receptor-Mediated Endocytosis: A Possible Mechanism of Viral Entry

Given that the AIDS virus binds to the T4 molecule on the cell surface, we must next consider what mechanisms the virus employs to introduce its genetic material into the cytoplasm of the cell. Previous studies with enveloped viruses have defined two distinct pathways by which the virus can enter the cell (White *et al.*, 1983). One mechanism, exemplified by paramyxoviruses, involves direct fusion of the viral envelope with the cell membrane. A second mechanism, employed by orthomyx-oviruses, for example, involves the association of virus with a specific cell-surface receptor such that the virus-receptor complex undergoes endocy-tosis. After endocytosis, the virus, now present within endosomes, fuses with the limiting membrane of the endosome in order to enter the cytoplasm. This fusion event is thought to be mediated by structural changes in the viral coat proteins. Moreover, such changes depend on the low-pH environment of the endosome (White et al., 1983).

Two recent observations suggest that the complex of AIDS virus and T4 on the cell surface is internalized via endocytosis. First, preliminary observations by Seth Lederman and Leonard Chess at Columbia, using immunoelectron microscopy, demonstrate that in resting T lymphocytes, most of the T4 resides on the cell surface. On activation of T cells with phytohemagglutinin or phorbol esters, most of the T4 protein is now pres-ent within endocytotic vesicles in the cytoplasm. These observations sug-gest that when T4$^+$ T lymphocytes are exposed to AIDS virus, the vi-rus is carried into the endosome via its T4-receptor molecule. Second, if the AIDS virus is internalized with T4 in the endosome, the viral glycoprotein is likely to undergo a pH-induced alteration to permit fusion and release of viral RNA into the cytoplasm. We would therefore pre-dict that agents that deacidify endosomes would inhibit release of AIDS virus from endosomes and block viral infection. In preliminary experi-ments, we have demonstrated that ammonium chloride, a weak base that deacidifies endosomes (Marsh, 1984), inhibits AIDS virus infection in vitro.

Taken together, our studies suggest a mechanism of AIDS virus in-fection that initially involves the specific association of the AIDS virus with T4 molecules on the cell surface. This association does not require additional T-cell-specific molecules and can be demonstrated on both B lymphocytes and epithelial cell lines. The complex of T4 and AIDS vi-rus is then likely to be internalized in endosomes via receptor-mediated endocytosis. The virus can then fuse with the limiting membrane of the en-dosome, releasing the nucleocapsid into the cytoplasm. Viral replication does not appear to require the environment of a T lymphocyte, since ac-tive infection is also observed in both human T4$^+$ B lymphocytes and epithelial cell lines. In this manner, a T-lymphocyte surface protein thought to be important in mediating effector cell-target cell interactions has been exploited by a human lymphotropic virus to specifically target the AIDS virus to populations of T4$^+$ cells.

References

Barre-Sinoussi, F., Chermann, J. C., Rey, F., Nugeyre, M. T., Chamaret, S., Gruest, J., Dauguet, C., Axler-Blin, C., Vezinet-Brun, F., Rouzioux, C., Rozenbaum, W., and Montagnier, L., 1983, Isolation of a T lymphotrophic retrovirus from a patient at risk for acquired immune deficiency syndrome (AIDS), *Science* **220**:868–871.

Biddison, W. E., Rao, P. E., Talle, M. A., Goldstein, G., and Shaw, S., 1982, Possible involvement of the OKT4 molecule in T cell recognition of class II HLA antigens, *J. Exp. Med.* **156**:1065–1076.

Blue, M.-L., Daley, J. F., Levine, H., and Schlossman, S. F., 1985, Coexpression of T4 and T8 on peripheral blood T cells demonstrated by two-color fluorescence flow cytometry, *J. Immunol.* **134**:2281–2286.

Clapham, P., Nagy, K., and Weiss, R. A., 1984, Pseudotypes of human T-cell leukemia virus types 1 and 2: Neutralization by patients' sera, *Proc. Natl. Acad. Sci. U.S.A.* **81**:2886–2889.

Cone, R. D., and Mulligan, R. C., 1984, High-efficiency gene transfer into mammalian cells: Generation of helper-free recombinant retroviruses with broad mammalian host range, *Proc. Natl. Acad. Sci. U.S.A.* **81**:6349–6353.

Dalgleish, A. G., Beverly, P. C. L., Clapham, P. R., Crawford, D. H., Greaves, M. F., and Weiss, R. A., 1984, The CD4 (T4) antigen is an essential component of the receptor for the AIDS retrovirus, *Nature (London)* **312**:736–766.

Engleman, E. G., Benike, C. J., Grumet, F. C., and Evans, R. L., 1981a, Activation of human T lymphocyte subsets: Helper and suppressor/cytotoxic T cells recognize and respond to distinct histocompatibility antigens, *J. Immunol.* **127**:2124–2129.

Engleman, E. G., Benike, C., Glickman, E., and Evans, R. L., 1981b, Antibodies to membrane structures that distinguish suppressor/cytotoxic and helper T lymphocyte subpopulations block the mixed leukocyte reaction in man, *J. Exp. Med.* **154**:193–198.

Gallo, R. C., Salahuddin, S. Z., Popovic, M., Shearer, G. M., Kaplan, M., Haynes, B. F., Palker, T. J., Redfield, R., Oleske, J., Safai, B., White, G., Foster, P., and Markham, P. D., 1984, Frequent detection and isolation of cytoplasmic retroviruses (HTLV-III) from patients with AIDS and at risk for AIDS, *Science* **224**:550–503.

Hildemann, W. H., 1979, Immunocompetence and allogeneic polymorphism among invertebrates, *Transplantation* **27**:1–3.

Hood, L., Kronenberg, M., and Hunkapiller, T., 1985, T cell antigen receptors and the immunoglobulin supergene family, *Cell* **40**:225–229.

Kabat, E. A., Wu, T. T., Bilofsky, H., Reid-Miller, M., and Perry, H., 1983, *Sequences of Proteins of Immunological Interest*, U.S. Department of Health and Human Services, Washington, D. C., p. 281.

Klatzmann, D., Barre-Sinoussi, R., Nugeyre, M. T., Dauguet, C., Vilmer, E., Griscelli, C., Brun-Vezinet, F., Rouzioux, C., Gluckman, J. C., Chermann, J.-C., and Montagnier, L., 1984a, Selective trophism of lymphadenopathy associated virus (LAV) for helper–inducer lymphocytes, *Science* **225**:59–63.

Klatzmann, D., Champagne, E., Chamaret, S., Gruest, J., Guetard, D., Hercend, T., Gluckman, J.-C., and Montagnier, L., 1984b, T-lymphocyte T4 molecule behaves as the receptor for human retrovirus LAV, *Nature (London)* **312:**767–768.

Krensky, A. M., Reiss, C. S., Mier, J. W., Strominger, J. L., and Burakoff, S. J., 1982, Long-term human cytolytic T-cell lines allospecific for HLA-DR6 antigen are OKT4[+], *Proc. Natl. Acad. Sci. U.S.A.* **79:**2365–2369.

Landegren, U., Ramstedt, U., Axberg, I., Ullberg, M., Jondal, M., and Wigzell, H., 1982, Selective inhibition of human T cell cytotoxicity at levels of target recognition or initiation of lysis by monoclonal OKT3 and Leu-2a antibodies, *J. Exp. Med.* **155:**1579–1584.

Littman, D. R., Thomas, Y., Maddon, P. J., Chess, L., and Axel, R., 1985, The isolation and sequence of the gene encoding T8: A molecule defining functional classes of T lymphocytes, *Cell* **40:**237–246.

Maddon, P. J., Littman, D. R., Godfrey, M., Maddon, D. E., Chess, L., and Axel, R., 1985, The isolation and nucleotide sequence of a cDNA encoding the T cell surface protein T4: A new member of the immunoglobulin gene family, *Cell* **42:**93–104.

Marrack, P., Endres, R., Schimonkevitz, R., Zlotnik, A., Dialynas, D., Fitch, F., and Kappler, J., 1983, The major histocompatibility complex-restricted antigen receptor on T cells. II. Role of the L3T4 product, *J. Exp. Med.* **159:**1077–1091.

Marsh, M., 1984, The entry of enveloped viruses into cells by endocytosis, *Biochem. J.* **218:**1–10.

McDougal, J. S., Cort, S. P., Kennedy, M. S., Cabridilla, C. D., Feorino, P. M., Francis, D. P., Hicks, D., Kalyanaraman, V. S., and Martin, L. S., 1985, Immunoassay for the detection and quantitation of infectious human retrovirus, lymphodenopathy-associated virus (LAV), *J. Immunol. Meth.* **76:**171–183.

McDougal, J. S., Kennedy, M. S., Sligh, J. M., Cort, S. P., Mawle, A., and Nicholson, J. K. A., 1986, Binding of HTLV-III/LAV to T4[+] T cells by a complex of the 11OK viral protein and the T4 molecule, *Science* **231:**382–385.

Meuer, S. C., Schlossman, S. F., and Reinherz, E., 1982, Clonal analysis of human cytotoxic T lymphocytes: T4[+] and T8[+] effector T cells recognize products of different major histocompatibility complex regions, *Proc. Natl. Acad. Sci. U.S.A.* **79:**4395–4399.

Reinherz, E. L., and Schlossman, S. F., 1980, The differentiation and function of human T cells, *Cell* **19:**821–827.

Rogozinski, L., Bass, A., Glickman, E., Talle, M. A., Goldstein, G., Wang, J., Chess, L., and Thomas, Y., 1984, The T4 surface antigen is involved in the induction of helper function, *J. Immunol.* **132:**735–739.

Saito, H., Maki, R. A., Clayton, L. K. and Tonegawa, S., 1983, Complete primary structures of the E$_\beta$ chain and gene of the mouse major histocompatibility complex, *Proc. Natl. Acad. Sci. U.S.A.* **80:**5520–5524.

Saito, H., Kranz, D. M., Takagaki, Y., Hayday, A. C., Eisen, H. N. and Tonegawa, S., 1984, A third rearranged and expressed gene in a clone of cytotoxic T lymphocytes, *Nature (London)* **312:**36–40.

Sim, G. K., Yague, J., Nelson, J., Marrack, P., Palmer, E., Augustin, A., and Kappler, J., 1984, Primary structure of human T-cell receptor α-chain, *Nature (London)* **312:**771–775.

Scofield, V. L., Schlumpberger, J. M., West, L. A., and Weissman, I. L., 1982, Protochordate allorecognition is controlled by a MHC-like gene system, *Nature (London* **295**:499–502.

Snow, P. M., and Terhorst, C., 1983, The T8 antigen is a multimeric complex of two distinct subunits on human thymocytes but consists of homomultimeric forms on peripheral blood T lymphocytes, *J. Biol. Chem.* **258**:1475–1481.

Snow, P. M., Keizer, G., Coligan, J. E., and Terhorst, C., 1984, Purification and N-terminal amino acid sequence of the human T cell surface antigen T8, *J. Immunol.* **133**:2058–2066.

Snow, P. M., van de Rijn, M., and Terhorst, C., 1986, Association between the human thymic differentiation antigens T6 and T8, *Eur. J. Immunol.* (in press).

Swain, S. L., 1981, Significance of Lyt phenotypes: Lyt2 antibodies block activities of T cells that recognize class I major histocompatibility complex antigens regardless of their function, *Proc. Natl. Acad. Sci. U.S.A.* **78**:7101–7105.

Swain, S. L., 1983, T cell subsets and the recognition of MHC class, *Immunol. Rev.* **74**:129–142.

Thomas, Y., Rogozinski, L., Irigoyen, O. H., Friedman, S. M., Kung, P. C., Goldstein, G., and Chess, L., 1981, Functional analysis of human T cell subsets defined by monoclonal antibodies. IV. Induction of suppressor cells within the OKT4[+] population, *J. Exp. Med.* **154**:459–467.

Tonegawa, S., 1983, Somatic generation of antibody diversity, *Nature (London)* **302**:575–581.

White, J., Kielian, M., and Helenius, A., 1983, Membrane fusion proteins of enveloped animal viruses, *Q. Rev. Biophys.* **16**:151–195.

Wilde, D. B., Marrack, P., Kappler, J., Dialynas, D. P., and Fitch, F. W., 1983, Evidence implicating L3T4 in class II MHC antigen reactivity: Monoclonal antibody blocks class II MHC antigen specific proliferation, release of lymphokines, and binding by cloned murine helper T lymphocyte lines, *J. Immunol.* **131**:2178–2183.

Williams, A. F., Barclay, A. N., Clark, M. J., and Gagnon, J., 1984, Cell surface glycoproteins and the origins of immunity, in: *The Proceedings of the Sigrid Juselius Symposium* (L. C. Andersson, G. C. Gahmberg, and P. Ekblom, eds.), Academic Press, New York, pp. 125–138.

Yanagi, Y., Yoshikai, Y., Leggett, K., Clark, S. P., Aleksander, I., and Mak, T. W., 1984, A human T cell-specific cDNA clone encodes a protein having extensive homology to immunoglobulin chains, *Nature (London)* **308**:145–149.

14

Identifying the Determinants of Protein Function and Stability

ROBERT T. SAUER, HILLARY C. M. NELSON, MICHAEL H. HECHT, and ANDREW PAKULA

1. Introduction

Protein sequences encode the information required to form specific three-dimensional structures (Anfinsen, 1973), but it is still not possible to predict protein structure and function from sequence information alone. It is possible, however, to understand the relationship among the structure, function, and sequence of some proteins. Our laboratory has been using genetic and biochemical approaches to define the determinants of protein structure and function for two sequence-specific DNA-binding proteins, the cI repressor and Cro protein of bacteriophage λ. We have been able to identify residues that play key roles in maintaining the folded structures of these proteins and residues that allow these proteins to bind specifically to operator DNA. Our interest has also been focused on the factors that determine intracellular protein turnover, since many mutant Cro proteins, but not mutant cI repressors, are hypersensitive to degradation. In this chapter, we review these studies and describe how intragenic, second-site reversion has been used to identify amino acid substitutions that enhance protein function.

ROBERT T. SAUER, HILLARY C. M. NELSON, MICHAEL H. HECHT, and ANDREW PAKULA • Department of Biology, Massachusetts Institute of Technology, Cambridge, Massachusetts 02139.

2. Repressor and Cro Background

When bacteriophage λ infects *Escherichia coli*, its choice between lysogeny and lytic multiplication is influenced by the relative levels of repressor, the product of the *c*I gene, and Cro, the product of the *cro* gene (Johnson *et al.*, 1981; Gussin *et al.*, 1983). Repressor is essential for lysogenization; it blocks expression of early and lytic genes, including *cro*, and activates its own synthesis. Cro promotes lytic growth, primarily by inhibiting the expression of repressor. Both proteins act by binding to the same six operator DNA sites. The opposing physiological consequences of repressor and Cro action result from differences in their relative affinities for each of the operator sites.

2.1. Protein Structures

The λ Cro protein is a small protein (66 residues/monomer) that is active as a dimer. In the crystal structure, each monomer includes three strands of β-sheet, three α-helices, and an additional strand of β-sheet that stabilizes the dimer (Anderson *et al.*, 1981; Ohlendorf *et al.*, 1982). The major features of the crystal structure are retained by Cro in solution (Weber *et al.*, 1985).

The λ repressor is a larger protein (236 residues/monomer) that is also active as a dimer. The monomer contains an N-terminal domain (residues 1–92), a hinge region (residues 93–131), and a C-terminal domain (residues 132–236) (Pabo *et al.*, 1979). DNA binding is mediated by the N-terminal domain (Sauer *et al.*, 1979). In the crystal structure, the N-terminal domain contains five α-helices (Pabo and Lewis, 1982). Helices 1–4 form a globular structure, while helix 5 interacts with helix 5′ from another monomer to form the dimer interface. Nuclear magnetic resonance studies indicate that the solution structure is similar to the crystal structure whether the N-terminal domain is free or part of intact repressor (Weiss *et al.*, 1983, 1987a). Structural information is not available for the C-terminal portions of λ repressor.

2.2. Complexes with Operator DNA

Models for the Cro–operator complex and the repressor–operator complex have been proposed on the basis of computer model-building studies (Anderson *et al.*, 1981; Ohlendorf *et al.*, 1982; Pabo and Lewis, 1982; Lewis *et al.*, 1983). In both cases, the models are supported by a large body of chemical protection data and genetic information (for a review, see Pabo and Sauer, 1984). Both proteins belong to the helix–turn–helix family of sequence-specific DNA-binding proteins; Cro's α-helix 3 and repressor's α-helix 3 serve analogous functions as the major recognition helices. These α-helices fit into the major groove of the operator, where hydrogen bonds and van der Waals interactions between side chains and base pairs provide much of the specificity of operator recognition. In Cro, other DNA interactions are mediated by side chains from α-helix 2 and the C-terminal β-region. In repressor, α-helix 2 and the N-terminal "arm" mediate additional DNA contacts. The "arm" wraps around the DNA to contact bases in the major groove on the back of the operator site (Pabo *et al.*, 1982).

3. Isolation of Phenotypically Defective Mutants

The system outlined in Fig. 1 can be used to isolate mutations in either the λ *cro* gene or the λ *cI* gene. If a plasmid directs the synthesis of active Cro or λ repressor, the protein binds to operator DNA and blocks expression of β-galactosidase from a chromosomal λ P_R–promoter-*lacZ* fusion. By contrast, if inactive Cro or repressor is synthesized, P_R is not turned off and β-galactosidase is expressed. In a system of this type, mutations will be detected only if they cause a sufficiently large decrease in the activity or level of the mutant protein. To avoid the isolation of mutations that have only minor effects, we overexpress the Cro and repressor proteins at levels about 100-fold higher than their derepression thresholds. This ensures that most mutations cause a 100-fold or greater decrease in the level or activity of the mutant proteins.

Following random mutagenesis, we identified λ Cro$^-$ or λ repressor$^-$ transformants by screening for lac$^+$ colonies (Hecht *et al.*, 1983; Nelson *et al.*, 1983; Pakula *et al.*, 1986).We then sequenced the structural gene and promoter region to determine the position and type of each mutation. In the Cro case, we sequenced 189 independent mutant candidates and found each to be altered by the substitution, deletion, or insertion of a single base pair. A few mutations were isolated five to eight times and probably represent mutagenic hot spots; most mutations were isolated

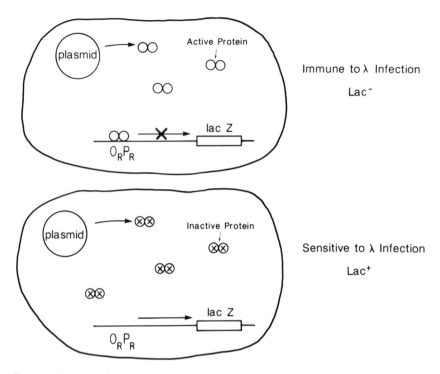

Figure 1. Screen for inactive λ repressor or λ Cro proteins. In the upper cell, the plasmid directs the synthesis of active protein, which binds to the operator and turns off *lacZ* expression. This cell is also immune to superinfection by phage λ. The mutant protein in the lower cell cannot bind operator DNA. This cell is Lac+ and sensitive to superinfection.

one to three times. The complete collection contains 83 different Cro⁻ mutations. Of these, 2 are frameshift mutations, 9 are promoter or ribosome binding mutations, 6 are nonsense mutations, and 66 are missense mutations. Figures 2A and 3A show the distributions of the missense and suppressed nonsense mutations in the protein sequences of Cro and the N-terminal domain of λ repressor. The distributions of the mutant sites in the wild-type protein structures are shown in Figs. 2B and 3B. In both cases, mutations occur throughout the protein sequence and structure. In Cro, the mutations affect 34 of the 66 residue positions; in the N-terminal domain of repressor, the mutations affect 26 of 92 residue positions. The genetic map of missense mutations is not saturated in either case. For ex-

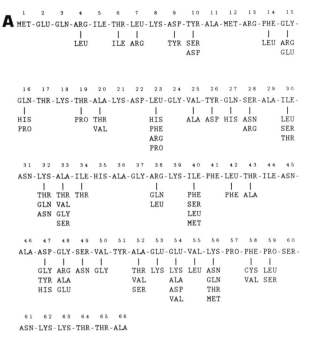

A

```
  1    2    3    4    5    6    7    8    9   10   11   12   13   14   15
MET - GLU - GLN - ARG - ILE - THR - LEU - LYS - ASP - TYR - ALA - MET - ARG - PHE - GLY -
                   |              |    |              |    |                        |    |
                  LEU            ILE  ARG            TYR  SER                      LEU  ARG
                                                         ASP                           GLU


 16   17   18   19   20   21   22   23   24   25   26   27   28   29   30
GLN - THR - LYS - THR - ALA - LYS - ASP - LEU - GLY - VAL - TYR - GLN - SER - ALA - ILE -
 |              |    |              |              |    |    |    |                   |
HIS            PRO  THR            HIS            ALA  ASP  HIS  ASN                 LEU
PRO                 VAL            PHE                           ARG                 SER
                                  ARG                                               THR
                                  PRO


 31   32   33   34   35   36   37   38   39   40   41   42   43   44   45
ASN - LYS - ALA - ILE - HIS - ALA - GLY - ARG - LYS - ILE - PHE - LEU - THR - ILE - ASN -
       |    |    |                   |              |              |    |
      THR  THR  THR                 GLN            PHE            PHE  ALA
      GLN  VAL                      LEU            SER
      ASN  GLY                                    LEU
           SER                                    MET


 46   47   48   49   50   51   52   53   54   55   56   57   58   59   60
ALA - ASP - GLY - SER - VAL - TYR - ALA - GLU - GLU - VAL - LYS - PRO - PHE - PRO - SER -
 |    |    |    |                   |    |    |    |    |              |    |
GLY  ARG  ASN  GLY                 THR  LYS  LYS  LEU  ASN            CYS  LEU
TYR  ALA                           VAL       ALA       GLN            VAL  SER
HIS  GLU                           SER       ASP       THR
                                             VAL       MET


 61   62   63   64   65   66
ASN - LYS - LYS - THR - THR - ALA
```

B

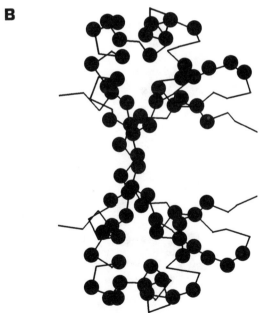

Figure 2. (A) Positions of missense mutations in the sequence of λ Cro. (B) Positions of missense sites in the structure of λ Cro are shown as solid black circles on the α-carbon backbone of the dimer.

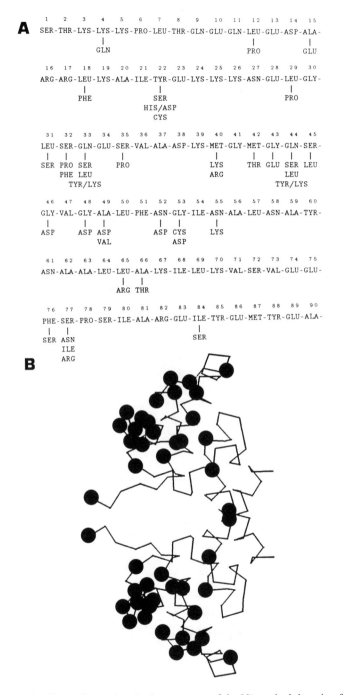

A

```
  1    2    3    4    5    6    7    8    9   10   11   12   13   14   15
SER-THR-LYS-LYS-LYS-PRO-LEU-THR-GLN-GLU-GLN-LEU-GLU-ASP-ALA-
                    |                        |        |
                   GLN                      PRO      GLU

 16   17   18   19   20   21   22   23   24   25   26   27   28   29   30
ARG-ARG-LEU-LYS-ALA-ILE-TYR-GLU-LYS-LYS-LYS-ASN-GLU-LEU-GLY-
              |         |                        |
             PHE       SER                      PRO
                    HIS/ASP
                      CYS

 31   32   33   34   35   36   37   38   39   40   41   42   43   44   45
LEU-SER-GLN-GLU-SER-VAL-ALA-ASP-LYS-MET-GLY-MET-GLY-GLN-SER-
  |   |   |       |                   |        |   |   |   |
 SER PRO SER     PRO                 LYS      THR GLU SER LEU
     PHE LEU                         ARG              LEU
     TYR/LYS                                          TYR/LYS

 46   47   48   49   50   51   52   53   54   55   56   57   58   59   60
GLY-VAL-GLY-ALA-LEU-PHE-ASN-GLY-ILE-ASN-ALA-LEU-ASN-ALA-TYR-
  |       |   |           |   |   |
 ASP     ASP ASP         ASP CYS LYS
             VAL             ASP

 61   62   63   64   65   66   67   68   69   70   71   72   73   74   75
ASN-ALA-ALA-LEU-LEU-ALA-LYS-ILE-LEU-LYS-VAL-SER-VAL-GLU-GLU-
                    |   |
                   ARG THR

 76   77   78   79   80   81   82   83   84   85   86   87   88   89   90
PHE-SER-PRO-SER-ILE-ALA-ARG-GLU-GLY-ILE-TYR-GLU-MET-TYR-GLU-ALA-
  |   |   |                       |
 SER ASN                         SER
     ILE
     ARG
```

B

Figure 3. (A) Positions of mutations in the sequence of the N-terminal domain of λ repressor. (B) Each mutant position is marked by a solid black circle on the α-carbon backbone of the protein dimer.

ample, several Cro⁻ mutations, at positions not represented in our collection, have been constructed synthetically (Caruthers *et al.*, 1986).

What can we conclude from the fact that missense mutations can be isolated at many different positions in repressor and Cro? The mutant side chains at these positions must block protein function in some manner, but this does not necessarily mean that the wild-type side chain is essential for function. Nevertheless, the sites of these mutations are clearly positions at which the chemical identity of the amino acid side chain is important. In other words, the side chains at these positions carry some information. The informational content is high if the wild-type side chain is the only functional residue, moderate if similar side chains are also functional, and low if almost all side chains are allowed. It is possible that some residue positions carry no functional information. Miller (1978, 1984) and his colleagues have surveyed a very large number of suppressed nonsense mutations in Lac repressor and have found that some positions can accommodate virtually any amino acid.

4. Structural Distribution of Mutant Sites

Since the wild-type crystal structures of λ Cro and the N-terminal domain of λ repressor are known (Anderson *et al.*, 1981; Pabo and Lewis, 1982), it is possible to ask about the structural distribution of the residues that are altered by missense mutations. For example, do most mutations affect solvent-exposed residues on the protein surface, or do they affect residues that are buried in the hydrophobic core? Of the 34 missense positions in Cro, 17 are relatively solvent-exposed and 17 are relatively buried. When total missense mutations are counted, the distribution is similar: 35 mutations change surface side chains and 31 alter buried side chains. The repressor mutations are distributed in the same fashion. In both cases, about half the mutations affect the protein surface and half affect the protein hydrophobic core.

For surface mutations, we can also ask whether the wild-type side chains are close to the operator DNA in the models of the protein–operator complexes. Figure 4 displays these results for Cro and repressor. In the N-terminal domain of λ repressor, all the sites of surface mutation lie close to the operator DNA. For Cro, many of the surface missense positions are close to the operator DNA, but a significant number are distant from the DNA.

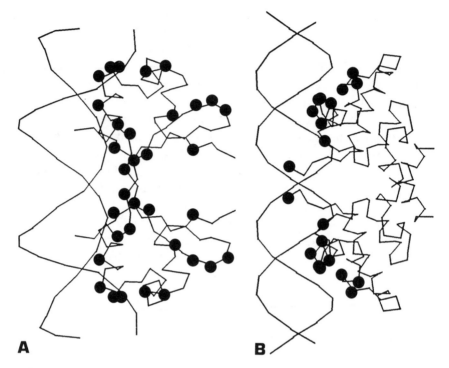

Figure 4. Positions of surface mutations in the protein–operator DNA complexes. (A) λ Cro. (B) λ Repressor.

5. Why Are Mutant Proteins Nonfunctional?

There are several ways in which a missense mutation could affect the binding of λ repressor or Cro to operator DNA. Some simple possibilities include:

1. The mutation might cause a decrease in the level of the mutant protein by increasing its sensitivity to intracellular proteolysis.
2. The mutant protein might be unfolded most of the time for thermodynamic reasons, or it might be unable to fold into the correct three-dimensional structure for kinetic reasons.
3. The mutant protein could be stably folded but unable to bind operator because a favorable operator contact had been removed or an unfavorable contact introduced.

The mechanisms are not exclusive; several may contribute to the phenotypic defects of particular mutant proteins.

5.1. Contribution of Proteolysis to Mutant Phenotypes

The distributions of the steady-state intracellular concentrations of the mutant proteins, relative to wild-type, are summarized in Fig. 5. The mutant λ repressor proteins are all present at or near wild-type levels (Hecht *et al.*, 1983; Nelson *et al.*, 1983). This is true even in cases in which the mutation affects the hydrophobic core of the protein.

A very different result is obtained for the mutant Cro proteins. Virtually all the proteins with mutations in the hydrophobic core and many of the proteins with surface mutations are present at levels that are less than 5% of the wild-type level. These severely reduced levels probably result from increased proteolysis, since pulse-chase experiments show that

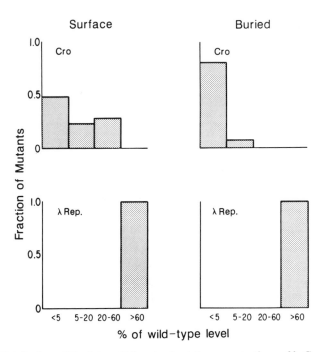

Figure 5. Distribution of the intracellular steady-state concentrations of λ Cro (*top*) or λ repressor (*bottom*) mutant proteins with surface substitutions (*left*) or buried substitutions (*right*).

the mutant proteins have turnover rates that are much faster than those of wild-type Cro (Pakula *et al.*, 1986). It is clear that the reduced levels of most of the mutant Cro proteins contribute to the phenotypic defects of these mutants. In fact, in some cases the defect is caused solely by the reduced intracellular level of the mutant protein. These mutant proteins have activities *in vivo* that are the same as the activity of wild-type Cro at a comparable concentration.

Why are most of the mutant Cro proteins hypersensitive to intracellular degradation? Since denatured proteins are proteolyzed much faster than folded proteins, a mutation could increase susceptibility to proteolysis by destabilizing the native structure and increasing the fraction of protein molecules in an unfolded state. In support of this idea, we find that almost all the mutant Cro proteins that are severely degraded have substitutions that would be expected to decrease the thermodynamic stability of the folded structure. These substitutions include changes in the tightly packed hydrophobic core, surface mutations that interfere with charge-stabilized hydrogen bonds, and mutations that replace glycines in tight turns with residues that cannot assume the same backbone conformation. The latter classes account for all the surface mutations that are distant from the DNA in the Cro–operator complex (see Fig. 4A).

5.2. Mutations That Affect Protein Stability

In the previous section, we suggested that the folded structures of many of the mutant Cro proteins are less stable than that of wild-type Cro. We have not been able to test this hypothesis because the levels of these mutant proteins are too low to allow purification. This is not a problem for the repressor mutants, and our biochemical efforts have concentrated on these proteins. As a first step, we purified mutant repressors with substitutions in surface or buried residues of the N-terminal domain and determined their thermal stabilities (Hecht *et al.*, 1984). Differential scanning calorimetry curves for several representative mutant proteins are shown in Fig. 6. The peaks near 70°C represent unfolding the C-terminal domains of wild-type and the mutant λ repressors. The wild-type N-terminal domain unfolds in a narrow range near 52°C. The Gln44 → Tyr surface mutation does not alter the thermal stability of the N-terminal domain. Most of the other N-terminal domains with surface substitutions were also found to have wild-type thermal stabilities. One exception is the N-terminal domain of the Gln33 → Tyr mutant (Fig. 6), which is ac-

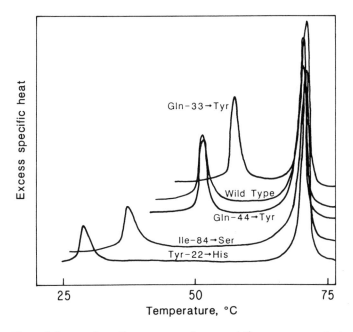

Figure 6. Thermal denaturation of λ repressor and representative repressor mutants as monitored by differential scanning calorimetry. The C-terminal domains of all the proteins denature near 70°C. The peaks between 25 and 60°C represent unfolding of the N-terminal domains of the wild-type and mutant proteins. The N-terminal domain of the Gln33 → Tyr mutant is more stable than wild-type.

tually more stable than wild-type! Computer modeling suggests that a new stacking interaction could occur between the mutant Tyr33 aromatic ring and a nearby ring. This may account for the increased stability of this mutant protein.

Some mutant repressors with substitutions in buried residues could not be purified. The N-terminal domains of these proteins are probably unfolded most or all of the time (unfolded proteins have poor solubility and can be lost by precipitation during purification). In those cases in which mutant proteins with buried substitutions could be purified, we found that the N-terminal domains were unstable but were folded at the low temperatures (4°C) used for purification. As shown in Fig. 6, the N-terminal domain of one of these proteins (Tyr22 → His) unfolds near 28°C, and that of another (Ile84 → Ser) unfolds near 37°C. Since the DNA-binding domains of both these proteins are substantially unfolded under physiological conditions, reduced stability clearly contributes to their reduced activity. The Ile84 → Ser mutant is also defective in assembly of the active dimer. This helix-5 mutation changes a residue that is part of the N-terminal dimer interface and reduces the dimerization constant by 100-fold or more (Weiss *et al.*, 1987b).

If λ repressor proteins with changes in buried residues are significantly or completely unfolded at 37°C, then why aren't these mutant proteins degraded rapidly in the cell? A possible answer is suggested by the observed concentration dependence of N-terminal unfolding *in vitro* (Hecht *et al.*, 1984). The thermal stability of the N-terminal domain decreases by about 7°C as the repressor concentration is increased, which can be explained if protein unfolding is accompanied by aggregation of the denatured chains. If aggregation also accompanies unfolding *in vivo*, proteolysis could be avoided in two ways. The aggregates could be soluble, but the unfolded chains might be poor substrates for proteolytic cleavage. Many proteases need to bind an extended region of the substrate polypeptide chain (Thompson and Blout, 1973), and such regions might not exist or be accessible in unfolded aggregates. Alternatively, the aggregates could be insoluble and form protease-resistant precipitates or complexes with membranes or other cellular components.

5.3. DNA-Binding Mutations

We define DNA-binding mutations using two operational criteria: First, the mutant protein must exist predominantly in the correct, folded structure under the conditions in which operator binding is measured. Second, the affinity of the mutant protein for operator DNA must be substantially reduced. For repressor, virtually all the surface mutations fall into this class. Moreover, since the sites of these mutations are close to the operator DNA in the proposed complex (see Fig. 4B), our operational definition seems reasonable. In Cro, those mutant proteins with moderate intracellular levels and very low activities fall in the DNA-binding class. As expected, the sites of these mutations also lie close to the operator DNA.

Some of the DNA-binding mutations affect residues that directly contact the operator DNA. For example, the Gln44 → Ser mutation of λ repressor removes two hydrogen bonds that normally form between the Gln44 side chain and an adenine in the major groove of the operator site. This mutation decreases operator affinity about 500-fold (Nelson and

Sauer, 1986). Other repressor mutations affect residues that are simply close to the operator. For example, the Gly43 → Glu mutation replaces a small side chain that is near the DNA with a larger, negatively charged side chain. The resulting steric or electrostatic repulsion decreases operator affinity 10,000-fold or more.

Most of the DNA-binding mutations reduce operator affinity without affecting the affinity of λ repressor for nonoperator sequences. This is true for the two mutations discussed above and for mutations such as Gln33 → Ser, which affect hydrogen bonds between the protein and the phosphate backbone of the operator DNA. For example, the Gln33 → Ser mutation causes a 2000-fold decrease in operator affinity, but only a 1.2-fold decrease in the affinity for nonoperator sites (Nelson and Sauer, 1986). This implies that the Gln33 side chain does not hydrogen bond to the sugar–phosphate backbone of a nonoperator site. It is possible that such a bond cannot form because steric interference (between side chains and bases in the major grooves) prevents close approach of the repressor to the nonoperator site. By this model, the Gln33–backbone hydrogen bond contributes to specificity because it can form only at sites, such as the operator, where there is a close fit of the van der Waals surface of the protein to that of the DNA.

A few of the DNA-binding mutations that alter the net charge of λ repressor do affect binding to nonoperator DNA. The Ala49 → Asp and Asn52 → Asp mutations decrease nonoperator affinity, while the Asn55 → Lys mutation increases nonoperator affinity. Overall, it seems likely that the repressor–nonoperator DNA complex is a rather loose structure that is stabilized by medium-range electrostatic interactions but lacks any detailed complementarity of van der Waals surfaces. This would explain why mutations that disrupt short-range operator interactions such as hydrogen bonds or van der Waals interactions do not affect binding to nonoperator DNA.

6. Phenotypic Reversion

The activity of a mutant protein can often be rescued by substitutions that do not restore the wild-type amino acid sequence. These substitutions can occur at the position of the original mutation (same-site revertants) or at other positions in the protein (second-site revertants). To obtain revertants of mutations in λ repressor's N-terminal domain, we subjected mutant plasmids to a second round of random mutagenesis and selected for repressors that could prevent lytic growth of phage λ (Hecht and Sauer, 1985; Nelson and Sauer, 1985). Because the mutant or revertant repressors are overexpressed, proteins can pass the selection even when their activity is less than that of wild-type.

6.1. Same-Site Revertants

Table I shows a number of same-site revertants of mutations in λ repressor's N-terminal domain (Hecht and Sauer, 1985). In some cases, the nature of the original mutant defect can be deduced from the properties of the revertant. For example, the Gly48 → Asp mutation in α-helix 3 is reverted by replacing the Asp with Asn. Since Gly48 is a surface residue that is close to the operator DNA, the mutant defect could have been caused by steric or electrostatic interference or both. However, the mutant Asp and revertant Asn side chains are sterically similar, indicating that the mutant defect is caused by electrostatic repulsion between the protein and DNA. In another surface case, the Ser35 → Pro mutation in α-helix 2 is reverted by replacing Pro with either Thr or Leu. This suggests that the inactivity of the Pro35 mutant results not from loss of the wild-type Ser, but rather from the insertion of Pro into an α-helical region of the protein. The information carried by residues 35 and 48 of λ repressor must be reasonably low, since revertant side chains can be accommodated at these positions even when their properties are quite different

Table I. Repressor Same-Site Revertants

Location	Wild-type		Mutant		Revertant		Activity at 37°C
α-Helix 1, buried	Tyr22	→	Ser22	→	Phe22	→	Dec. 15-fold
α-Helix 2, surface	Ser35	→	Pro35	→	Leu35	→	Inc. 3-fold
	Ser35	→	Pro35	→	Thr35	→	Wild-type
α-Helix 3, surface	Gly48	→	Asp48	→	Asn48	→	Inc. 3-fold
Loop-4, buried	Ser77	→	Asn77	→	Cys77	→	Dec. 50-fold
	Ser77	→	Asn77	→	Thr77	→	Wild-type

from those of wild-type. It seems likely that this will also be true at many other surface positions in the protein.

The side-chain requirements for buried residues are more restricted. For example, substitution of the buried Tyr22 residue with Ser, Cys, Asp, or His reduces the stability of the N-terminal domain and results in a mutant phenotype. The Phe22 revertant differs from wild-type only in its lack of the phenolic hydroxyl group, but this small difference is sufficient to cause a 15-fold reduction in activity (Table I). Surprisingly, the N-terminal domain of the Phe22 revertant is slightly more stable than wild-type (Hecht *et al.*, 1985). Reduced stability therefore cannot account for its lowered activity. We presume that the Tyr22 → Phe change causes a subtle alteration in the protein structure. The Tyr22 hydroxyl group appears to hydrogen-bond to the protein backbone near α-helix 2, which is one of the DNA-binding helices. It is possible that helix 2 in the Phe22 revertant assumes a slightly different position with respect to the operator DNA.

Another buried residue, Ser77, participates in a charge-stabilized hydrogen bond with Asp14. Mutants with Asn77, Ile77, or Arg77 are inactive; a revertant with Cys77 has low activity; and a revertant with Thr77 has full activity (Table I). Since Cys is sterically similar to Ser but is a poor former of hydrogen bonds, we ascribe the low activity of the Cys77 revertant to the loss of the wild-type hydrogen bonds. We assume that the Thr77 revertant is fully active because Thr can form hydrogen bonds that are equivalent to those formed by Ser. Taken together, these results suggest that the charge-stabilized hydrogen bond between the side chains of residues 14 and 77 is an important determinant of repressor stability.

6.2. Second-Site Revertants

Some λ repressor mutations are reverted by sequence changes, called second-site "suppressor" mutations, that occur elsewhere in the protein (Table II) (Hecht and Sauer, 1985; Nelson and Sauer, 1985). The Gly48 → Ser and Glu34 → Lys changes suppress several primary mutations, the Glu83 → Lys change was isolated as a suppressor of one mutation, and the Val36 → Ile change was isolated only in combination with the Glu34 → Lys suppressor mutation. In general, the second-site suppressors do not fully restore wild-type activity. This is illustrated in Fig. 7, which shows *in vivo* activity as a function of temperature for a mutant protein bearing zero, one, or two suppressor mutations. The Glu34 → Lys

Table II. Repressor Second-Site Revertants

Mutation	Location		Suppressor	Location
Lys4 → Gln	Arm/surface	+	Glu34 → Lys	Helix 2/surface
		+	Gly48 → Ser	Helix 3/surface
		+	Glu83 → Lys	Helix 5/surface
Ala15 → Glu	Helix 1/buried	+	Gly48 → Ser	Helix 3/surface
Ser35 → Pro	Helix 2/surface	+	Glu34 → Lys	Helix 2/surface
		+	Gly48 → Ser	Helix 3/surface
Ser77 → Asn	Loop 4/buried	+	Glu34 → Lys	Helix 2/surface
		+	Glu34 → Lys	Helix 2/surface
			Val36 → Ile	Helix 2/buried

suppressor increases the activity of the Ser77 → Asn mutant, and the Val36 → Ile suppressor increases the activity further. However, the protein bearing the primary and both suppressor mutations is as active as wild-type only at 30°C. At higher temperatures, the triply substituted repressor is less active than wild-type.

6.3. Suppression Occurs by Enhancement of Activity

In principle, second-site suppressors might act to correct mutant defects in an allele-specific fashion or to overcome defects by improving protein function or stability in a global fashion. In the latter case, the second-site substitution should confer on an otherwise wild-type protein activity or stability that is greater than that of wild-type. To test this possibility, we cloned the Glu34 → Lys, Gly48 → Ser, and Glu83 → Lys second-site changes into wild-type backgrounds and purified the corresponding repressor proteins (Nelson and Sauer, 1985). As shown in Fig. 8, each of the revertant substitutions increases the affinity of λ repressor for operator DNA. When compared with wild-type repressor, the Ser48 protein binds with 25-fold-increased affinity, the Lys83 protein with 80-fold-increased affinity, and the Lys34 protein with 600-fold-increased affinity. These results indicate that second-site suppression occurs, at least in part, through a global mechanism that involves improved binding to operator DNA.

The Gly48 → Ser change increases the thermal stability of the N-terminal domain by 4°C (Hecht *et al.*, 1985). This enhanced stability may contribute to its suppression of mutations such as Ala15 → Glu, which reduce the stability of the N-terminal domain. In such cases, the Ser48 sup-

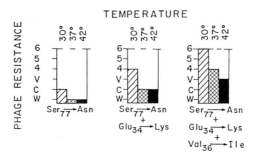

Figure 7. Activities *in vivo* of mutant and revertant λ repressor proteins as a function of temperature. The vertical scale represents the immunity to superinfection by clear or virulent derivatives of phage λ. Wild-type repressor mediates resistance to level 6, at each of the temperatures. Thus, the triply substituted repressor has activity comparable to wild-type only at 30°C.

pressor would increase the fraction of repressor molecules that were in the folded conformation and would increase the operator affinity of these folded molecules. Enhanced stability is unlikely to contribute to second-site suppression by the Glu34 → Lys or Glu83 → Lys changes, since these substitutions cause slight reductions in the thermal stability of the N-terminal domain.

For the Glu34 → Lys and Gly48 → Ser revertants, increased affinity appears to result from new interactions with the operator DNA. Figure 9 shows that the sites of these changes are quite close to the operator DNA. In addition, computer model-building suggests that the revertant side chains could engage in plausible interactions with the operator (Nelson and Sauer, 1985). The Lys34 side chain, in α-helix 2, can form an ion pair with a phosphate group on the operator backbone. This substitution was also found to substantially increase the affinity of repressor for nonoperator DNA, suggesting that a similar electrostatic interaction is possible with the backbone of a nonoperator site. In the cell, the increased operator and nonoperator affinity must balance each other, since the Lys34 protein has an activity that is very close to that of wild-type repressor. The Ser48 side chain, in α-helix 3, can hydrogen-bond to a phosphate oxygen on the operator DNA backbone. This substitution causes a small increase in nonoperator affinity, but the Ser48 protein is more active in the cell than is wild-type, suggesting that the change increases the specificity of operator recognition.

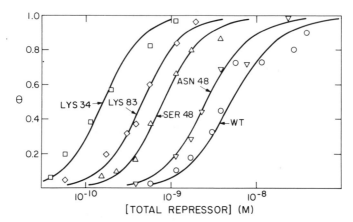

Figure 8. Binding of wild-type and revertant λ repressor proteins to DNA containing the O_R1 operator site. Binding was assayed by nitrocellulose filter binding of ^{32}P-labeled operator DNA.

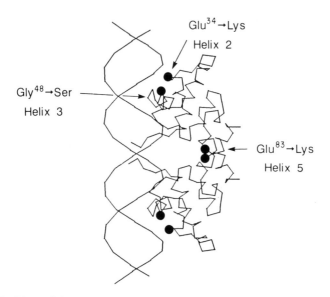

Figure 9. Positions of the Glu34 → Lys, Gly48 → Ser, and Glu83 → Lys second-site suppressor mutations in the protein–DNA complex.

The Glu83 → Lys suppressor mutation seems to increase operator affinity by a mechanism that is different from those of the Glu34 → Lys and Gly48 → Ser suppressors. Unlike these changes, the site of the Glu83 → Lys mutation is not close to the operator DNA (Fig. 9). This substitution does not increase the affinity of repressor for nonoperator DNA, and salt-dependence data show that the Lys83 side chain is not involved in a salt bridge with the operator. The site of the Lys83 substitution is close to the dimer contacts of the N-terminal domain, and it is possible that the revertant side chain stabilizes a tertiary or quaternary conformation that allows better overall contact with the operator site.

7. Summary

The reduced operator DNA-binding activity of the mutant λ repressor and λ Cro proteins can be attributed, in most cases, to one or more of the following causes:

1. Some mutations cause reductions in activity, but have little or no effect on protein stability. Most of these amino acid changes identify solvent-exposed side chains that directly mediate protein function. In the repressor and Cro cases, such residues form the DNA-binding surfaces of the proteins. A few of the mutations in this class result in conservative substitutions of buried side chains (e.g., Tyr22 → Phe in λ repressor). It seems likely that these substitutions cause small changes in the structure of the DNA-binding surfaces without causing substantial changes in the global structure of the protein.

2. Some mutations reduce thermal stability to the point where most protein molecules are in an unfolded and therefore inactive conformation. In our experience, such mutations account for a major fraction of all missense mutations. Most of these mutations change residues in the tightly packed hydrophobic core, where any substantial change would be expected to cause instability. Other ''stability'' mutations change surface residues involved in charge-stabilized, tertiary hydrogen bonds or glycines in tight turns. It seems likely that the wild-type residues at these positions are major determinants of protein folding and stability.

3. Some mutations increase the rate of intracellular proteolytic degradation and decrease the steady-state concentration of the mutant protein. In Cro, this phenotype correlates with reduced stability, and it seems likely that unfolded Cro molecules are good substrates for cellular proteases.

Unfolded repressor molecules are not proteolyzed in the cell, apparently because the unfolded chains aggregate.

Reversion analysis allows us to extend the information gained by studying mutant proteins. Same-site revertants provide information about the chemical and steric informational requirements at a given side-chain position. Second-site revertants, in the λ repressor case, identify amino acid changes that increase the affinity for operator DNA and, in some cases, increase thermal stability. We believe that the ligand-binding and stability properties of most proteins have not been maximized and that second-site reversion will provide a generally applicable method for improving protein function and stability.

ACKNOWLEDGMENTS. This work was supported by NIH Grants AI-16892 and AI-15707 and by a grant from W. R. Grace, Inc. We thank Brian Matthews and Carl Pabo for the coordinates of λ Cro and the N-terminal domain of λ repressor and Rob Campbell for help with computer graphics.

References

Anderson, W. F., Ohlendorf, D. H., Takeda, Y., and Matthews, B. W., 1981, Structure of the Cro repressor from bacteriophage λ and its interaction with DNA, *Nature (London)* **290:**754–758.

Anfinsen, C. B., 1973, Principles that govern the folding of protein chains, *Science* **181:**223–230.

Caruthers, M. H., Barone, A. D., Beltman, J., Bracco, L. P., Dodds, D. R., Dubendorff, J. W., Eisenbeis, S. J., Gayle, R. B., Prosser, K., Rosendahl, M. S., Sutton, J., and Tang, J. Y., 1986, The interaction of Cro, *c*I, and *Escherichia coli* RNA polymerase with operators and promoters, *J. Cell. Biochemistry* (in press).

Gussin, G., Johnson, A.D., Pabo, C. O., and Sauer, R. T., 1983, Repressor and Cro protein: Structure, function, and role in lysogenization, in: *Lambda II* (S. Stahl, J. Roberts, R. Hendrix, and A. Campbell, eds.), Cold Spring Harbor Press, Cold Spring Harbor, New York, pp. 93–121.

Hecht, M. H., and Sauer, R. T., 1985, Phage lambda repressor revertants: Amino acid substitutions that restore activity to mutant proteins, *J. Mol. Biol.* **186:**53–63.

Hecht, M. H., Nelson, H. C. M., and Sauer, R. T., 1983, Mutations in λ repressor's amino-terminal domain: Implications for protein stability and DNA binding, *Proc. Natl. Acad. Sci. U.S.A.* **80:**2676–2680.

Hecht, M. H., Sturtevant, J. M., and Sauer, R. T., 1984, Effect of single amino acid replacements on the thermal stability of the NH_2-terminal domain of phage λ repressor, *Proc. Natl. Acad. Sci. U.S.A.* **81:**5685–5689.

Hecht, M. H., Hehir, K. M., Nelson, H. C. M., Sturtevant, J. M., and Sauer, R. T., 1985, Increasing and decreasing protein stability: Effects of revertant substitutions on the thermal denaturation of phage λ repressor, *J. Cell. Biochem.* **29**:217–224.

Johnson, A. D., Poteete, A. R., Lauer, G., Sauer, R. T., Ackers, G. K., and Ptashne, M., 1981, Lambda repressor and Cro: Components of an efficient molecular switch, *Nature (London)* **294**:217–223.

Lewis, M., Jeffrey, A., Wang, J., Ladner, R., Ptashne, M., and Pabo, C. O., 1983, Structure of the operator-binding domain of bacteriophage λ repressor: Implications for DNA recognition and gene regulation, *Cold Spring Harbor Symp. Quant. Biol.* **47**:435–440.

Miller, J. H., 1978, The *lacI* gene: Its role in *lac* operon control and its use as a genetic system, in: *The Operon* (J. H. Miller and W. Rezhikoff, eds.), Cold Spring Harbor Press, Cold Spring Harbor, New York, pp. 31–88.

Miller, J. H., 1984, Genetic studies of the *lac* repressor. XII. Amino acid replacements in the DNA binding domain of the *Escherichia coli lac* repressor, *J. Mol. Biol.* **180**:205–212.

Nelson, H. C. M., and Sauer, R. T., 1985, λ Repressor mutations that increase the affinity and specificity of operator binding, *Cell* **42**:549–558.

Nelson, H. C. M., and Sauer, R. T., 1986, Interaction of mutant λ repressors with operator and non-operator DNA, *J. Mol. Biol.* (in press).

Nelson, H. C. M., Hecht, M. H., and Sauer, R. T., 1983, Mutations defining the operator binding sites of bacteriophage λ repressor, *Cold Spring Harbor Symp. Quant. Biol.* **47**:441–449.

Ohlendorf, D. H., Anderson, W. F., Fisher, R. G., Takeda, Y., and Matthews, B. W., 1982, The molecular basis of DNA-protein recognition inferred from the structure of Cro repressor, *Nature (London)* **298**:718–723.

Pabo, C. O., and Lewis, M., 1982, The operator-binding domain of λ repressor: Structure and DNA recognition, *Nature (London)* **298**:443–447.

Pabo, C. O., and Sauer, R. T., 1984, Protein-DNA recognition, *Annu. Rev. Biochem.* **53**:293–321.

Pabo, C. O., Sauer, R. T., Sturtevant, J. M., and Ptashne, M., 1979, The lambda repressor contains two domains, *Proc. Natl. Acad. Sci. U.S.A.* **76**:1608–1612.

Pabo, C. O., Krovatin, W., Jeffrey, A., and Sauer, R. T., 1982, The N-terminal arms of λ repressor wrap around the operator DNA, *Nature (London)* **298**:441–443.

Pakula, A., Young, V., and Sauer, R. T., 1986, λ Cro mutations: Effects on activity and intracellular degradation, *Proc. Natl. Acad. Sci. U.S.A.* (in press).

Sauer, R. T., Pabo, C. O., Meyer, B. J., Ptashne, M., and Backman, K. C., 1979, Regulatory functions of the lambda repressor reside in the amino terminal domain, *Nature (London)* **279**:396–400.

Thompson, R. C., and Blout, E. R., 1973, Dependence of the kinetic parameters for elastase-catalyzed amide hydrolysis on the length of peptide substrates, *Biochemistry* **12**:57–65.

Weber, P. L., Wemmer, D. E., and Reid, B. R., 1985, ^{1}H NMR studies of λ Cro repressor. 2. Sequential resonance assignments of the ^{1}H NMR spectrum, *Biochemistry* **24**:4553–4562.

Weiss, M. A., Karplus, M., Patel, D. J., and Sauer, R. T., 1983, Solution NMR studies of intact lambda repressor, *J. Biomol. Struct. Dynam.* **1**:151–157.

Weiss, M. A., Karplus, M., and Sauer, R. T., 1987a, The ^{1}H-NMR aromatic spectrum of the operator-binding domain of the λ repressor: Resonance assignment with application to structure and dynamics, *Biochemistry* (in press).

Weiss, M. A., Pabo, C. O., Karplus, M., and Sauer, R. T., 1987b, Dimerization of the operator-binding domain of phase λ repressor, *Biochemistry* (in press).

Index